Allow Me!

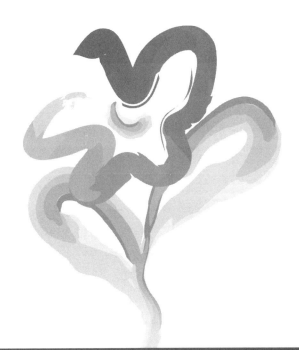

A Guide to Promoting Communication Skills in Adults with Developmental Delays

IRMA D. RUITER

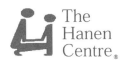
The
Hanen
Centre

Allow Me

by Irma Ruiter

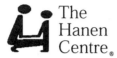

The
Hanen
Centre®

Copyright © 2000 by Hanen Early Language Program

National Library of Canada
ISBN 0-921145-15-2

Copies of this book may be ordered from the publisher:

THE HANEN CENTRE

1075 Bay Street, Suite 515
Toronto, Ontario
Canada M5S 2B1

Telephone: (416) 921-1073
Fax: (416) 921-1225
e-mail: info@hanen.org
web: www.hanen.org

Illustrations: Lily Con
Editors: Elaine Weitzman and Vilia Cox
Book Design: Dave Murphy/ArtPlus Design & Communications
Book Layout: Barb Neri/ArtPlus Design & Communications

Allow Me is a publication of the Hanen Early Language Program and was supported by funding from the Ontario Ministry of Community and Social Services.

Printed in Canada by The Beacon Herald Fine **Printing Division.**

Acknowledgements

I would like to extend my heartfelt thanks to all those people who have supported the production of this guidebook for the benefit of adults with developmental delays.

This guidebook would not have been possible without funding from the Ontario Ministry of Community and Social Services, Toronto Area Office. I would like to thank Frank Cummings, who was The Hanen Centre's Ministry Program Supervisor at the time, for his tremendous support of this project.

Ayala Manolson is my inspiration and mentor in this project and I am deeply thankful for her belief in this application and in me.

Thank you to the staff of The Hanen Centre, especially Tom Khan, who have had to put up with draft after draft of this book, and who have been valuable liaisons between me and others in different parts of the country. I appreciate their personal interest, their warmth and their readiness to assist, which they have always extended to me. I would especially like to thank Elaine Weitzman for editing the completed manuscript and Vilia Cox for reviewing Elaine's edits.

I wish to thank Marianne Becker and Diane Nunziato for their valuable contributions to the guidebook, and Katie Zartman, Linda Moroz and Wanda McCullogh for their insight and input into the program.

Much thanks to the Board and Management of Bethesda Programs who gave me the opportunity to try something new and to share it with others.

To my parents, Ted and Trudy Ruiter, and my siblings — Yvonne Scott, Ron Ruiter, Shirley House and Cynthia Koudijs — and to my friends, Joan Buchner and Danielle Reynolds, goes my appreciation for their love, encouragement and support, with which I was able to keep going and to keep my perspective.

Most of all, I extend my personal appreciation to every single person in Niagara and Toronto who participated in the "Allow Me" Program over the last 10 years — it is their feedback and support that have encouraged its development, defined the shape of the program and nurtured its growth. They continue to do so today.

To David Madore and Brian Smith — always in my heart.

Table of Contents

A Note on the Use of "He" and "She"

For simplicity's sake, this book refers to conversation partners in the male gender in Chapters 1, 3, 5 and 7 and in the female gender in Chapters 2, 4 and 6. The exceptions occur when there are examples in these chapters of partners of specific genders.

This does not apply to examples which are either illustrated or which are described in narrative format.

How We Define "Facilitator"

The use of the term "facilitator" in this book recognizes the number of significant people in the lives of adults with developmental delays, who support and promote their interaction and communication so they can participate fully in their communities. These facilitators may be parents or other family members; educational, residential or vocational staff; friends or other people who are involved in the day-to-day lives of people with developmental delays.

The term "facilitator" in no way refers to the use of "Facilitated Communication" and in no way reflects this method of intervention.

Introduction

Each of us has a need to be touched by another person. We long for relationships in which we are known, understood and loved for who we are. Who we are is communicated by what we do and what we say. How well we are known depends on how well others actually listen to and observe us; how well we are understood depends on how others interpret our words and actions; how well we are loved depends on how accepting others are of us. This is not a one-way street: we, too, must do our share in knowing, understanding and loving others. This is one of the things that give meaning to our lives – that there is someone else out there whom we can touch deeply and who can touch us.

People with developmental delays, like the rest of us, are eager to reveal who they are. Like the rest of us, who they are evolves over time – they too can grow and change in their human journey. All this requires some form of language. But often people with developmental delays don't talk the way you and I do, so it can be harder for us to get to know them, to discover their interests, dreams and heartbreaks. And so it can be harder to teach them the language they need. More than usual then, communication becomes a barrier: when people are frequently misunderstood, they learn to stop reaching out, or to reach out in ways that lead to more misunderstanding.

This guidebook is offered as one way in which we can connect with people who have developmental delays — in a way in which language can be nourished, and in which the wonder and beauty of each person is revealed.

Irma Ruiter

Chapter One Slow Down and Capture the Moment

All human beings need to communicate, to let others know their needs, feelings, opinions and desires. But many people with developmental disabilities have difficulty telling us what they want to say. These people's lives are restricted by their limited ability to communicate, and those of us who spend time with them may know little about what they need, feel and think. People with developmental delays, however, *can* become better communicators and more active members of their communities, but they can't do it alone. What they need are skilled, responsive communication partners who can help them share their feelings and thoughts. When this happens, they will become *our* conversation partners.

Part of becoming a better conversation partner involves being able to communicate spontaneously without being pushed or prompted. However, before an individual is willing to initiate an interaction, he must feel confident that his messages will be responded to. This is easier said than done with unsophisticated communicators, whose messages are easy to miss or misinterpret.

If an individual is to learn to communicate effectively, communication must be a powerful tool in his life. The power of communication is felt only when his messages are heard and responded to. Such a response builds a feeling of trust, security and confidence, a sense of connection with the rest of the world — something many of us take for granted.

In this chapter, you will:

- discover how caring connections help your partners learn the power of communication

- discover what you can realistically expect from your partners when they communicate with you

- become familiar with your partners' interests and with those times that are best for encouraging communication

EVERYONE COMMUNICATES IN SOME WAY

Although your partner may not speak, he communicates in other ways. He uses his own unique combination of body language, sounds, gestures, objects, pictures, signs and words. As his conversation partner, you may be aware of some of the ways he communicates, but you may not understand much of what he is trying to tell you.

Because a person's sense of the power of communication comes from being understood, your task is to become more skilled at recognizing and understanding what your partner is telling you.

To become aware of your partner's communication, take the time to:

S hare activities

L isten to what your partner is saying

O bserve your partner's behaviour

W ait — give your partner a chance to communicate

SLOW DOWN

Share activities

You can focus more clearly on your partner's communication skills when the two of you are doing something together. There are many times during the day when you shop, cook, eat, clean house, do laundry and have fun together. Doing things together provides you with a framework within which you can, **observe** and **wait** for your partner to communicate; at the same time, you can note **how** and **why** he is communicating with you.

Listen to what your partner is saying

Listen to your partner's words and sounds. Even if your partner cannot speak, the length of his sounds as well as their intonation, stress and pitch, provide important clues about the way he is feeling or what he wants to tell you. A short, sharp, loud sound may convey anger; a quiet hum that varies gently in pitch may convey satisfaction; a loud, persistent sound can also be used to get attention. Each individual's use of sounds is meaningful to him — and it is your job to interpret them.

Observe your partner's behaviour

You receive a great deal of information about a person when you watch what he does. Observe your partner's **facial expressions, gestures, direction of eye gaze, body position** when around certain items and activities, and his **general level of participation and alertness** during the activity. Based on his reactions, what might your partner be telling you? Take note of the **time of day** in which he appears to be more alert than others. Is there a pattern? Be aware of the **objects** he handles, and what he does with them.

Examine the environment. Watch for your partner's reactions to:

Sound — such as the noise of several people in a group or even of a specific person who is with the two of you, or the building's sounds such as fans and the hum of electrical wires or fluorescent lighting.

Touch — a light touch, such as a caress on his head or handling certain material like clay, or a deeper touch, such as a firm hand-hold while crossing a busy street, may be either irritating or pleasant to your partner.

Smell — his reaction to odours, such as your perfume or shampoo, can send you messages about his interests, likes or dislikes.

Lighting — your partner may be calmer in natural daylight or incandescent lighting rather than fluorescent, or in dimmer environments rather than brighter ones.

Take the time to observe your partner's behaviour closely. His actions can tell you many things that he cannot tell you with words. The messages which you tune into through examining the environment can help make the environment more comfortable for your partner and encourage even more communication to occur.

Wait — give your partner a chance to communicate

We tend to be very efficient people. When the doorbell rings, we answer it; when milk is spilled, we wipe it up; when our partner needs his coat, we get it for him. When we think our partner might want or need something, we anticipate what it is and provide it for him. We are often unaware that our efficiency deprives our partner of those vital opportunities to ask for or to comment on something.

The simple act of **waiting** will allow your partner to demonstrate that he is more capable of sending messages than you think. **Allow him to surprise you!** Waiting may encourage your partner to use a sign, say a word or make a gesture he has seldom used before.

There are other benefits to waiting. People with developmental delays cannot respond to what is said to them as quickly as we can. First, they must grasp what has been said to them; then they must think about how to respond. The problem is that they are rarely given the time to complete this cycle. Because we don't give them enough time to respond, they don't always realize that a response is expected of them. Some even learn to ignore what is said to them. But when you say something to your partner and then wait, he learns that he is **expected** to respond. The cycle of frustrated communication is broken, and you benefit too — you no longer have to work so hard to get that response!

Waiting for someone to communicate is very difficult. It requires real effort and lots of practice. But the payoffs are great. You will reap the reward when you find your partner approaching you more often to "talk" to you!

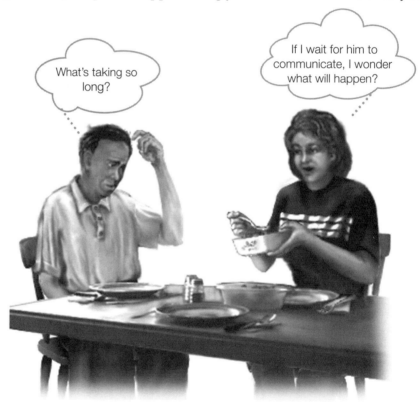

Bev decides to wait before she serves Gus to give him a chance to make a request.

Gus imitates signs but never seems to use them spontaneously. When Bev, his facilitator (please refer to page 6 for a definition of "facilitator"), thinks Gus wants something, she either gives it to him right away or she models the sign that she *wants him to produce. One day at dinner, she decides to give him a chance to communicate for himself. Rather than dishing out the food, she asks Gus what he wants, and then waits for him to respond. Gus is used to being served without being asked what he wants, and so he does not respond immediately. But when Bev waits, Gus realizes that he isn't going to be served in the usual way. He also realizes that he is expected to let her know what he wants; so after a few confused moments, he signs "eat". And then he is served very promptly!*

By ALLOWing Gus the opportunity to communicate for himself, Bev discovers that he is far more capable than she had originally thought.

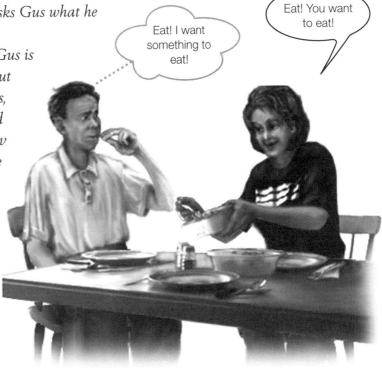

Bev is rewarded with the sign for "eat"!

THE HANEN LEVELS OF COMMUNICATION

Level 1 – Your partner's communication is reflexive

Level 2 – Your partner does not send messages intentionally, but you are able to read his body language

Level 3 – Your partner sends messages intentionally, using a combination of sounds, gestures and eye gaze

Level 4 – Your partner intentionally sends messages, using symbols such as words, signs, pictures

Level 5 – Your partner uses sentence fragments

Level 6 – Your partner uses simple sentences

Level 1 – Your partner's communication is reflexive

At first, your partner sends you messages about his wants, needs and interests through his reflexive behaviour. He does this unintentionally. He has no thought about getting his message across to you — it is you who assigns meaning to the message, and you respond *as if* it were communicative.

At this level, you interpret your partner's:

- cries
- looks
- startles
- smiles
- screams
- vowel-like sounds
- skin tone changes
- voice changes (loudness, pitch, intonation)
- body movements and/or position changes

Tara sits in a wheelchair all day long. She loves music. We know this because she smiles and laughs when music is played, and her smile fades when the music stops. She also laughs when things amuse her, and she cries when she is hungry or over-stimulated. Her facilitators know when she is hungry because she opens her mouth to be fed. When she is no longer hungry, she clamps her mouth shut. Sometimes she cries for no apparent reason and these sobs are loud and lonely. It is up to her facilitator to figure out what Tara feels or wants. Sometimes that's hard to do. ❦

At Level 1, Tara sends messages through reflexive behaviour, with no intent to communicate with others.

Level 2 – Your partner does not send messages intentionally, but you are able to read his body language

At this level, your partner does not deliberately direct messages to you, but he is more aware of you and sends messages that are consistent and easier to interpret. While he may enjoy spending time with you and may communicate frequently when he is with you, intentionality (communication with a specific goal in mind) is not yet established.

In addition to communicating in ways described in Level I, your partner communicates through:

- facial expressions
- reaching/moving toward an object
- vocalizing, using a variety of consonant and vowel sounds
- focusing on an object/person
- such actions as pushing away an unwanted item or reaching for something he wants

At Level 2, messages are beamed into the atmosphere like radio signals, and it is our job to pick them up!

Shelly does not talk, and the only sounds heard from her are cries or laughs. During meals, she always tosses her cup over her shoulder onto the floor. Traditionally, Shelly's facilitators have considered this a behaviour problem and handled it by helping her pick up the cup, often through hand-over-hand prompting.

At lunch time one day, Shelly's facilitator brings a loaf of bread and a jar of peanut butter to the table where Shelly is sitting. She shows the bread and peanut butter to Shelly, who looks at them and smiles. The facilitator, reassured that this is what Shelly wants to eat, takes the bread and peanut butter to the counter to make Shelly's sandwich. Immediately, Shelly tosses her cup onto the floor.

For Shelly, "out of sight" means "gone." She thinks she isn't going to get what she wants and she communicates her frustration by tossing the cup. This is her only way of responding to an uncertainty she must have felt for a long time. Because the action is not directed at anyone in particular, her facilitators do not see it as communicative. 🌿

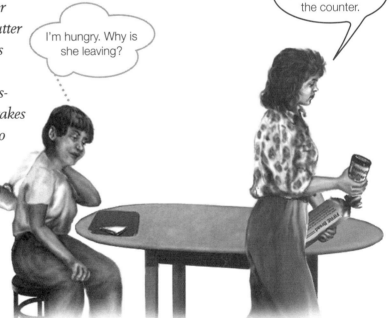

Shelly, a Level 2 communicator, isn't sure her facilitator is coming back with lunch. In her anxiety, she tosses her drink.

Level 3 – Your partner sends messages intentionally, using a combination of sounds, gestures and eye gaze

Your partner understands that if he needs or wants something, he has to communicate it directly to you — a clear indication of intentional communication. He may be able to say a few words or use a few signs, but mostly he sends messages purposefully through sounds and body movements.

At this level, your partner communicates by:

- looking directly at you
- pulling you to what he wants or bringing what he wants to you
- pointing, gesturing — e.g., nodding, waving
- using pantomime — e.g., pretending to smoke
- using sounds that stand for words
- occasionally using single words or signs
- combining eye gaze, vocalization (sounds) and gestures

Susan's facilitators encourage and expect her to use sign language to communicate. They are puzzled, however, because every time she wants something, Susan produces a whole series of signs. For example, when she wants yogurt, she signs, "coffee, milk, help, eat, please." This results in confusion, with Susan's facilitators trying to guess what she wants, and with Susan clarifying her request through gestures and by reaching for or pushing away what she is offered.

In frustration, the facilitators take a good look at what Susan does and at how they respond to her. This helps them realize that she does not yet understand that each sign has a special meaning. Instead, she considers signs to be a series of actions she has to perform in order to get something. Her real message — "I want yogurt, not milk" — is in her body language, and her facilitators respond better to that than to the many "signs" she uses.

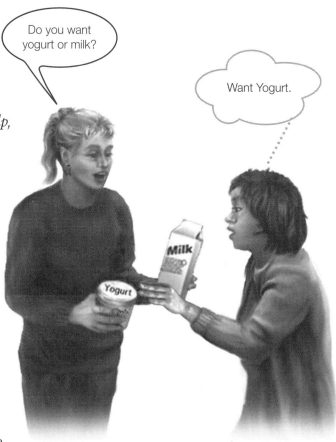

At Level 3, Susan's message is communicated intentionally and clearly through her actions.

Level 4 – Your partner intentionally sends messages, using symbols such as words, signs and pictures

Your partner consistently uses words, picture symbols or signs. He is able to understand more of what is said to him, but he continues to understand language better in the here-and-now. He can participate in conversation fairly readily, and he is able to respond with a wider variety of words and word combinations.

At this level, he communicates by:

- using single words or signs
- combining words (although these may be hard to understand)
- combining two words or signs in phrases/sentences.

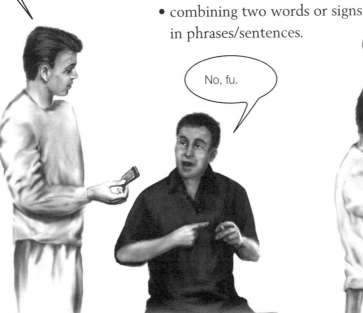

Mario, a Level 4 communicator, often mixes English and Italian.

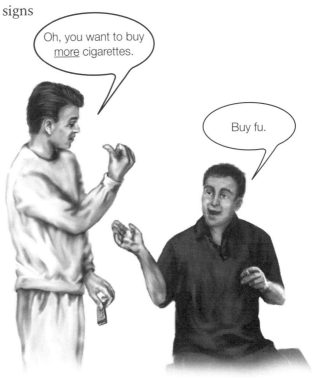

Alex has finally figured out that many of Mario's sentences are a mixture of Italian and English.

Mario's parents are immigrants who speak little English. Mario has several words and part-words in his repertoire, many of which are English and many of which are variations on words in his parents' language. He speaks in simple words and in two-word combinations. His speech is impaired and this impairment, together with his ethnic words and part-words, makes him hard to understand. He tries to supplement his speech with gestures, but even these consist largely of pointing in the general direction of "somewhere out there." He needs augmentative communication; however, his preferred way of communicating is through speech, and his primary facilitator has figured out many of his words and sounds.

One day Mario's facilitator, Alex, finds Mario with an unlit cigarette in his hand and an anxious look on his face. When Alex offers to light the cigarette, Mario says, "No, fu." Alex knows that "fu" is short for the Italian word for to smoke, "fumare" and that this is Mario's last cigarette in his package. "Fu" then is Mario's request to buy more cigarettes. 🌾

Level 5 – Your partner uses sentence fragments

Your partner is able to combine words, picture symbols or signs into two- to four-word phrases and incomplete sentences. He may continue to be hard to understand, and his speech may still be supplemented with gestures and body language. Conversations are likely to be most successful when they are based on his (as opposed to your) focus. At this level, your partner may give the impression of understanding almost everything that is said to him.

*K*atie has spent most of her life in an institution, where she is heavily sedated. As a result, she rarely speaks. When she moves into a group home, sedation is discontinued, and the staff find her eager to learn. She enjoys it when her facilitator puts make-up on for her and is able to give specific directions as to how she wants it applied. She tells her facilitator "Lip-ik lip", "That on cheek" and "Powder on nose". Her facilitator is pleasantly surprised at Katie's progress, especially when she is able to "tune in" to what interests her.

Level 6 – Your partner uses simple sentences

This individual is able to put four or more words together into short sentences that are basically grammatically correct. However, his listeners may still have trouble understanding him. He may leave smaller words out of sentences, such as "at", "to", "the", but the gist of what he is trying to say is understandable. He may have trouble figuring out how to talk about things that have occurred in the past or will occur in the future; instead, he continues to speak as if such events are occurring in his life at the present time. Pronouns may still be confusing to him, and he may refer to the same person as "he" and "she". He doesn't realize that you don't know the people he does, and he may refer to them, forget to identify them by name, or refer to them only as "he" or "she" when he first begins to talk about them. His stories aren't sequenced, and details are missing. His speech may still make it hard to understand the words he is saying.

*A*lphonse has Down Syndrome and is a very friendly and chatty young man. He is able to converse, and offers information and answers questions easily. This past winter, he flew to Florida from Toronto for a vacation with two facilitators and three peers. Two months after his return, he met a new friend and was able to tell him about the holiday in sentences like "There was so many people. All guys from Cuba. All in States."

At what level or levels does *your* partner communicate?

WHY AND HOW YOUR PARTNER COMMUNICATES

It often takes real skill to decipher your partner's message — an ability that develops through trial and error. Taking the time to WAIT, OBSERVE and LISTEN will help you discover two important things:

- **WHY** your partner communicates
- **HOW** your partner communicates

In the past, we have focused most of our attention on *how* developmentally delayed people communicate. If they could not talk, we gave them picture boards, taught them signs, or even tried to teach them some words. Despite all our efforts, they were slow to adapt to these forms of communication. Sometimes they weren't ready. Sometimes we failed to realize that our focus was much too narrow. We were teaching our partners to **request** what they wanted or to **label** an object — only two of the many, many reasons for which language is used.

Several reasons for communicating are listed below under the heading "WHY Your Partner Communicates". Read the list and beside each WHY, describe HOW your partner communicates for this purpose. Use the behaviours listed under "The Hanen Levels of Communication" as a guide and add any other information that describes your partner's level of communication.

WHY Your Partner Communicates	**HOW** Your Partner Communicates
Shows that he is aware of others by	_____
Protests/refuses/rejects by	_____
Accepts what is offered by	_____
Draws attention to things, people or events going on around him by	_____
Requests something by	_____

WHY Your Partner Communicates	**HOW** Your Partner Communicates
Requests routines and activities (e.g., stands beside the car to signal he wants a ride) by	_____
Expresses feelings by	_____
Greets by	_____
Comments (provides information on a topic — e.g., "I like your shirt," "It's hot today", or accompanies an action — e.g., "Up you go") by	_____
Asks you to do something for him by	_____
Communicates choices by	
Questions by	_____
Points out mistakes by	_____
Offers help by	_____
Asks for clarification (if unsure of what was said) by	_____
Other	_____

The above list does not give all the reasons why people communicate. As you observe and listen to your partner, you may discover that he communicates for other reasons.

WHEN YOUR PARTNER COMMUNICATES BEST

Your partner may communicate with you more at some times than at others. He may be most eager to communicate when he first arrives home from work in the afternoon, immediately following an exercise class in the evening or during breakfast in the morning. Consider WHEN your partner communicates best.

My partner communicates best:

In the morning when . . .

In the afternoon when . . .

In the evening when . . .

At weekends when . . .

WHAT INTERESTS YOUR PARTNER?

When we are involved in something that interests us, our attention is focused and we are eager to learn. We become motivated to learn the skills (including language) that are part of the activity, and we usually enjoy the company of the people who share it with us.

Ask yourself what your partner enjoys doing in his spare time. Below are four different categories of experiences, one or more of which your partner may enjoy. These are the kinds of experiences that you can use to hook your partner's interest and motivate him to learn from you.

Coming up with answers may be easy for some of your partners. However, it may be more difficult to think of activities that appeal to others because some people with developmental delays just don't seem to have interests. These people simply observe activities around them or ignore them entirely. For them, it is important that you be extra sensitive. SLOW down (Share, Listen, Observe and Wait) and look for activities that seem to attract their attention. Note where they go, what they look at, touch and vocalize at, as well as observing their skin tone and other subtle cues. Sharpening your observation and listening skills can help you tune into experiences that offer you the greatest potential to interact with your partners.

Early sensory experiences

Sensory experiences of this kind represent one of the least advanced ways in which a person amuses himself. He uses his senses of sight, sound, smell, touch and taste by:

- putting things in his mouth
- tapping items on surfaces
- crinkling paper in his ear
- chewing items such as food or paper
- sniffing people's hands or clothes
- rocking his body (for the vestibular stimulation)
- draping himself around stereo speakers or washing machines to experience the vibration

The individual who engages in sensory stimulation usually has his own agenda and rarely engages another person in the activity.

Does this describe your partner?   YES ☐   NO ☐

My partner's specific interests that fall into this category include:

_____

_____

Daily routines

Routines take many different forms for people with developmental delays. One type of routine involves completing a certain set of activities at the end of the day. For example, after work one person may always take a bath and then have supper, while another person will always make a complete tour of the house before settling down. As their facilitator, you aren't necessarily involved in these daily routines — and heaven help you if you interfere with them!

Other routines open themselves to more interaction. These are activities that occur on a daily, weekly or monthly basis when the person is involved with:

- personal grooming, conducted in the same order every day
- playing the same games over and over
- watching the same TV show or listening to the same music
- performing specific work duties
- telling the same stories over and over again
- daily chores

Does this describe your partner?   YES ☐   NO ☐

My partner's specific interests that fall into this category include:

_____

_____

_____

Community excursions

Your partner enjoys many of the activities we tend to take for granted, such as:

- shopping
- going to the movies or to the library
- going through car washes
- picking berries during fruit season
- parties
- visiting
- camping
- attending hockey games and other sporting events

Does this describe your partner?   YES ☐   NO ☐

My partner's specific interests that fall into this category include:

_____

_____

Creating

Your partner is able to be creative with his time and talents.

Your partner may be able to include others in his activity, but he can also be creative on his own. What he does create may not be sophisticated, not how you think it should be done; but it's his idea and no one else's, and he can be proud of it!

He may also imitate conventional activities, such as typing on the computer or playing baseball. He may even come up with new ways of doing things with these items — for example, he may roll a baseball bat back and forth to you or use it to roll a ball on the floor!

Does this describe your partner?   YES ❑   NO ❑

My partner's specific interests that fall into this category include:

_____

_____

_____

_____

Favourite recreational activities

Your partner enjoys *doing* things either by himself or with others. For example:

- going for walks
- riding a motor bike
- checking under the hood of a car
- taking things apart
- mowing the grass
- sports — watching or playing
- art

In general, if the activity keeps your partner actively involved in some way, you can be fairly sure that it's a special interest of his.

Does this describe your partner?   YES ❑   NO ❑

My partner's specific interests that fall into this category include:

_____

_____

_____

_____

LET'S REVIEW

For your partner to learn to communicate effectively, you must be aware of the many ways in which he sends messages. You must first:

SLOW down your interactions:

S hare activities

L isten to what your partner is saying

O bserve your partner's behaviour

W ait — give your partner a chance to communicate

Your partners all function at different levels and have varying levels of confidence in their ability to get a response from you. In order to adapt your behaviour to each of your partners, you must know their level of communication.

- Level 1   Your partner's communication is reflexive
- Level 2   Your partner does not send messages intentionally, but you are able to read his body language
- Level 3   Your partner sends messages intentionally, using a combination of sounds, gestures and eye gaze
- Level 4   Your partner intentionally sends messages, using symbols such as words, signs, pictures
- Level 5   Your partner uses sentence fragments
- Level 6   Your partner uses simple sentences

People use language for many reasons, and persons with developmental delays are no exception. It is important to focus not only on HOW a person communicates but also on WHY he does so. If a person has no reason to communicate, how he communicates won't matter much.

When your focus is on trying to encourage your partner to communicate, it is also essential to know the time of day at which he is most alert and willing to be with you, and the activities in which he prefers to engage. Taking advantage of these opportunities can help secure your partner's attention and promote more learning. Your partner may prefer the following types of activities:

- early sensory experiences
- daily routines
- community excursions
- creating
- favourite recreational activities

Chapter Two Allow Your Partner to Lead

Communication is a dynamic, interactive process, shaped by the interplay between the people who are communicating. What one person says to another and how she says it will affect what the other person says and how *she* says it. For example, if Jean asks Brenda a question, Brenda will probably answer it. However, if Jean shares some information about herself, Brenda might respond with a comment or a question about what Jean has said. And if Jean shouts at Brenda, Brenda may respond either by shouting back or by just walking away.

Most people take their ability to interact with others for granted. Years of successful, enjoyable interactions enable them to expect nothing less. Sadly, people with developmental delays are unlikely to have experienced the same success; as a result, they lack confidence in their ability to communicate. Success, however, is not beyond their reach. With your help, your partners *can* experience successful communication — when you allow them to lead.

To allow your partners to lead, you must create many, many opportunities for them to communicate. And when they do communicate, your responses should enable them to experience **successful** communication. Allowing your partners to lead may involve forgetting your "agenda", *giving up* the lead and changing your expectations. While this can be difficult, it's encouraging to know that, in so doing, you are engineering interactions which can have a significant and positive impact on your partners' lives.

In this chapter, you will:

- identify the roles you play during interactions with your partners — roles which can affect their opportunities to learn and communicate

- learn that your partners have different conversational styles, which affect how they interact with you

- learn how to allow your partners to lead and how to be a more responsive conversation partner

- learn how to follow your partners' lead by applying strategies that promote interaction and language learning

THE ROLES YOU PLAY MAKE A DIFFERENCE

Caregivers of people who are vulnerable have to take on a number of different roles. At various times you may find yourself in the role of helper, mover, teacher and friend. When you interact with a partner who has difficulty communicating, the kind of role you play will have an enormous impact on how well and how often she communicates, as well as on how much she learns.

When you play the "Helper" role . . .

It's natural to want the people you care for to be content and comfortable. Sometimes, however, this desire translates into an intensive effort to fulfill your partner's every need. Your "Helper" instincts may make things simpler, easier and faster, but they also deprive your partner of many, many opportunities to express her needs, wants and feelings. As a result, she learns that she does not *need* to communicate.

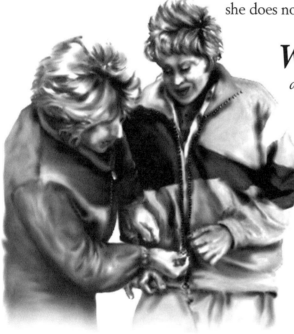

Heather is so intent on getting Molly ready to go home, she doesn't give her a chance to ask for help.

*W*hen Molly's facilitator (Please refer to page 6 for a definition of "facilitator"), Heather, completed the checklists in Chapter 1, she described Molly's communication as being typical of a partner at Level 3. Molly is Heather's favourite client, and they enjoy many routines together. One of these routines occurs at the end of the day when it's time for Molly to go home. In the winter, Heather helps Molly open her locker and put on her coat and boots. She always zips Molly's jacket up for her because she knows that Molly can't do this herself. When Molly is ready to leave, Heather takes her outside and helps her into the van. As the "Helper", Heather misses about seven opportunities to allow Molly to communicate. 🌸

When you play the "Mover" role . . .

When you work with adults who have developmental delays, every day is busy. You probably have many different duties to perform, schedules to follow and not enough time for everything. In an effort to keep up, it's easy to become a "Mover", and to allow communication to take second place to keeping up with duties and schedules. In the "Mover" role, you might find yourself talking at your partner rather than *with* her. You might even postpone conversations so you can meet your deadlines. This is especially true when you are working with several partners at once. Meals and other routines can become hectic, with little time to spare for small talk.

*P*atrick has had an exciting day at work and wants to tell John, his facilitator, about it. However, four other people are clamouring for dinner, and he can't get a word in edgeways. Later, the dishes are done, two people have gone shopping and one has gone to night school. But now that there's a moment in the evening to talk, Patrick has forgotten what he wanted to say. The moment for connecting with him has been lost.

The "Helper" and the "Mover" are always busy!

If something:
> breaks . . . . they fix it
> falls . . . . they pick it up
> is not there . . . . they go and get it
> is off . . . . they turn it on
> is on . . . . they turn it off
> is open . . . . they close it
> is out of reach . . . . . . they get it

When you play the "Director" role . . .

In the "Director" role, you see yourself as a teacher and organizer. Whether the activity involves household chores, recreational activities or doing something relaxing like flipping through photographs, in the "Director" role, you take control. You might find yourself using (or even overusing) commands and questions to ensure that your partners communicate or perform activities according to your expectations. And you will usually find yourself doing most of the talking, which can be overwhelming for many of your partners. When interactions are overwhelming, your partners tend to communicate less and less. Even when they *do* communicate, it is easy to miss their tentative attempts if you're not listening and watching for them.

*J*oe communicates at Level 2. When he is thirsty, he reaches for a glass of juice which Steven, his facilitator, places in front of him. Although Joe is not yet ready to use signs, Steven tries to get him to produce the sign for "drink". On one occasion, Steven says "Sign 'drink', Joe" 33 times in a row to try to get him to use the sign! But Joe shows what he wants by reaching for the juice. In his "Director" role, Steven does not respond to Joe's clear message and delays giving him the drink he wants so badly. Joe withdraws and engages in self-stimulation, which the frustrated Steven then attempts to discourage.

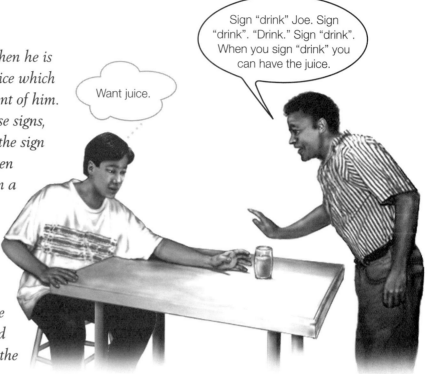

In the role of "Director", it's easy for Steven to miss or ignore Joe's communication.

It is difficult to know what your partner is ready to learn when your attention is focused on teaching and directing. **If you do more directing than interacting, your partner can't develop the confidence he needs to become an independent, competent communicator.**

When you play the "Responsive Conversation Partner" role . . .

Communication and language skills flourish when you play the "Responsive Conversation Partner" role. In this role, you watch to see what your partner is interested in and you wait for her to communicate. Your response depends on the messages she sends. This is where two-way communication comes in — your response to your partner's message lets her know that her communication has been successful. As she continues to experience successful communication, she becomes motivated to keep trying.

"Responsive Conversation Partners" try to help only when help is really needed, to make time for conversation even when they are busy and to let their partners lead the interaction. It's not easy being a "Responsive Conversation Partner", but it makes interaction easier and more fun for your partner.

*W*illiam *uses gestures, body language and some single words to communicate. When he says "Ba" and heads for his huge physiotherapy ball, his facilitators, Brad and Emily, count to three with him and wait for him to say "Up". When he says it, they repeat "Up" and then boost him onto the ball. When William wants the ball to roll, he begins to move his body and Brad and Emily gently rock the ball. From time to time, they pause so he can let them know whether or not he wants to continue. When William slides off the ball during one of these pauses, they know he wants to stop. His facilitators' sensitivity and responsiveness allow William to lead, enabling him to let them know what he enjoys and when he has had enough. He is then able to avoid the overstimulation that could result from less alert and responsive facilitators.*

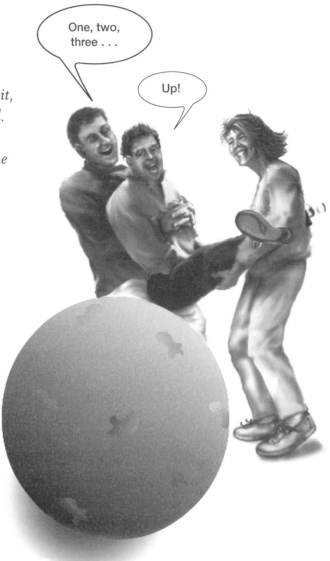

As "Responsive Conversation Partners", Brad and Emily build in opportunities for William to communicate during the activity, and when he communicates, they respond appropriately.

REMEMBER . . . it takes two to talk, and what you do with your half of the conversation makes all the difference. There will always be times when you have to play the "Helper", the "Mover" or the "Director" roles, but be aware that these roles make it hard for your partner to become a better communicator. When you spend most of your time in the "Responsive Conversation Partner" role, you **create** many more opportunities for your partner to learn to communicate.

THE FOUR CONVERSATIONAL STYLES

It isn't always easy to be a "Responsive Conversation Partner". While some of your partners may be eager to interact with you, others may resist your efforts to engage them. Some partners may approach you, while others may go so far as to avoid you. It all depends on their conversational style.

Your partner's conversational style is determined by her ability and motivation to **initiate** interactions with others and to **respond** when they initiate toward her. Some people are better at initiating than responding; some are better at responding than initiating; and some are equally competent at both. The section below illustrates four different conversational styles that arise from a combination of abilities to initiate and respond.

The partner with her own agenda

A partner with **her own agenda** may initiate, but it's usually because she wants something. She seldom initiates just for the sake of interacting with you, but if she does, her initiation may have nothing to do with the ongoing activity or topic of discussion. It tends to be very difficult to get a person with her own agenda to respond to *your* initiations.

The partner with a reluctant conversational style

A partner with a **reluctant** conversational style usually responds when you initiate an interaction, although she may need time to "warm up". However, she seldom initiates an interaction with you unless she really wants something or knows you very well. A partner with a reluctant conversational style can usually communicate more frequently and better than she typically does.

The partner with a passive conversational style

A partner with a **passive** conversational style seldom initiates or responds and seems unable to understand much of what is said. This makes it difficult for others to reach her.

The partner with a sociable conversational style

A partner with a **sociable** conversational style enjoys interacting with others and initiates and responds equally well.

Not everybody falls neatly into specific conversational styles. Overlaps or shifts into different styles occur as a result of personality, mood, time of day, familiarity with the environment and people, and so on. Your challenge is to recognize your partner's predominant style so you know how to allow her to lead.

ALLOW YOUR PARTNER TO LEAD BY ENCOURAGING HER TO INITIATE

If your partner's conversational style makes it difficult for you to interact with her, she needs to be encouraged to **initiate** interactions. You do this by holding back, by waiting to see what interests her and by giving her a chance to communicate while you remain silent, listening and watching intently. In this way, you **allow her to lead**.

In order to allow your partner to lead, you have to identify what her lead is. Some of your partners with reluctant or passive conversational styles may seldom initiate. However, if you observe them closely, you will pick up more initiations than you might expect.

It is especially important to:

- Wait
- Observe; and
- Listen to your partner

Your partner's messages can be very subtle — a change in facial expression, a quick look, a small hand movement, a soft sound or a slight movement of the body. These can be momentary and quickly lost. Be on the lookout for any of your partner's behaviours that send you messages — and respond to these **immediately**.

If, however, your partner doesn't give you many openings — create some. This is especially important when your partner has her own agenda; you may need to set up an activity that is interesting enough to hold her attention, no matter how briefly. Once she has been engaged by you, she will initiate because she will want the interaction to continue.

Lyle, at Level 2, has his own agenda. He likes to sit and rock with his fingers in his mouth, ignoring others' attempts to draw him into activities. Laura, his facilitator, knows that one of his few interests is having his hands rubbed with hand lotion. She decides to do this to capture his attention. While rubbing his hands, she pauses and waits. Lyle suddenly stops rocking, which lets Laura know that he is aware of what she is doing and that she has stopped! When she resumes rubbing his hands, Lyle resumes rocking. She has his attention!

When your goal is to allow your partner to lead during interactions, you must look for ways to engage her or be engaged by her. With this focus in mind, you will find a way to make that connection.

FOLLOW YOUR PARTNER'S LEAD

Once your partner has initiated or shown you what she is interested in, then you **follow her lead**.

There are three tried-and-true techniques for following your partner's lead:

- Respond immediately
- Interpret — say it as your partner would if she could
- Imitate what your partner says and does

Follow your partner's lead: RESPOND immediately

People who are developmentally delayed learn in ways that are very concrete. They connect events that happen close together in time and they have difficulty making this connection if there is too great a time lag between two events.

This principle is especially important with regard to communication. Prompt responses to her initiations help your partner see the connection between her behaviour and yours, whereas delayed or inconsistent responses make this difficult. If your partner makes a sound and looks at you and you take five seconds to respond, she won't realize that your response is connected to the sound she made. Thinking that she was not responded to, she may try again, she may give up or she may become angry and lash out. Sometimes a behaviour problem is simply your partner's way of responding to this unpredictability.

Your partner needs an **immediate and prompt response** to her communication in order to learn cause-and-effect. When you follow her lead and respond to her, she learns to connect your positive response to her behaviour and she experiences the power of communication. This makes it well worth her while to keep trying to get her messages across.

*P*olly *communicates at Level 3. She laughs, rocks and chatters incessantly, but much of her behaviour seems unconnected to what is happening around her. She requests things infrequently (using body language), seems to look through people and doesn't mind if you stay or if you leave. She has an* *intention tremor and her fine motor skills are poor. Her facilitators are trying to tune in to her behaviour so they can figure out the meaning of her messages and respond to them promptly.*

Polly's facilitator, Shawn, has given her a choice between two activities, and Polly has chosen to listen to her favourite music on tape. She tries to insert the cassette into the tape recorder, but she can't. Shawn resists the temptation to be the "Helper" and waits with an expectant look on his face. Finally, Polly hands the cassette to him. Shawn immediately slips it into the machine, but he doesn't close the dust cover. He waits to see if she will communicate a second time.

Polly tries to close the cover but her intention tremor makes it difficult. She takes Shawn's hand and pulls it toward the machine, and Shawn immediately closes the dust cover, saying, "Close it. You want me to close the cover."

Polly has initiated twice in a matter of minutes and Shawn knows that his patience and willingness to wait have enabled her to do this. In addition, Shawn realizes that his prompt responses have helped Polly learn something fundamental — that if she communicates, she can count on him to respond. ✿

Stay tuned — there's more to this story on page 38.

By responding promptly to your partner's initiations, you allow her to experience successful communication, which is the best and most natural reinforcement for the act of communication!

When responding to your partner, it's important to be willing to "go with the flow" and to adapt to what your partner is interested in. If you don't, your partner may lose out on some wonderful learning experiences.

Natalie, who is a bright Level 4 communicator, can say only a few words. Most of the time, she communicates using a picture board.

Brian is Natalie's facilitator, and today he and Natalie are getting together for a coffee break. Brian has Natalie's picture board in front of her and has made sure that the pictures she might need for this activity are available. All the items they need are on the table.

Brian is usually the one who pours the coffee, but today he holds back so that Natalie can ask for a cup of coffee using her picture board. Natalie realizes that she has to make a request and begins to scan her picture board. However, her finger passes the picture for coffee and stops at "cookie". Brian's first impulse is to say, "No, ask for coffee, Natalie". But he checks himself and responds to Natalie's unexpected initiation saying, "Cookie! You want a cookie!" and offers her one. By "going with the flow" and offering Natalie what she wants, Brian has enabled her to experience successful communication. ✿

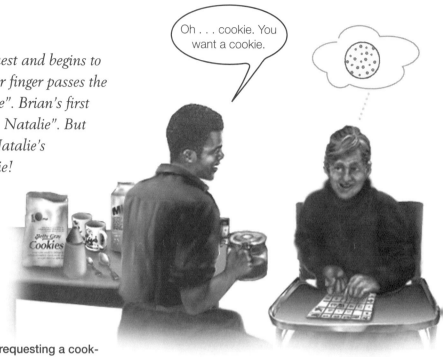

Natalie surprises Brian by requesting a cookie when he expected her to ask for coffee. By "going with the flow" and responding to her unexpected initiation, Brian enables Natalie to experience successful communication.

REMEMBER . . . Communication is a two-way street. Prompt responses to your partner's initiations, whether or not these initiations are intentional, are the best reinforcement your partner can get. If communication works the first time, she'll try again.

Follow your partner's lead: INTERPRET — say it as your partner would if she could

You can't always comply with your partner's wants. Other demands may compete for your attention or the desired item or activity may be unavailable or unsafe. However, your **interpretation** of your partner's intention will still provide her with the acknowledgment that her message has been received.

Interpret your partner's non-verbal message by "translating" it into words. Think of this as "pasting" spoken language over the message your partner sends with her eyes, her body language and her sounds.

Your responsive interpretations will:

- confirm your interest in your partner's message
- let your partner hear the verbal equivalent of her message
- give your partner a chance to correct you if you are wrong
- promote your partner's understanding of language

Your translation, however, must be at her level in order for her to learn from it.

For example:

When your partner points to a book that has fallen onto the floor, you can interpret by saying, "The book FELL!"

If she makes a face when eating, you can interpret by saying, "You don't like the carrots!"

REMEMBER... It is through this constant pairing of your partner's nonverbal communication and your verbal interpretation that her comprehension, and in time, her ability to express herself, will grow.

Merv is a likeable young man, who communicates intentionally using body language (Level 3). He is on a special diet and his snacks always come to work with him in his own cookie tin. One day his facilitator, Sharon, tries to persuade him to give her one of his cookies. Merv smiles and looks at Sharon, whose hand is open and outstretched. Then he slyly drops a plastic-wrapped piece of cheese into her hand. Sharon looks at it, laughs and says, "You don't want to give me a cookie! You (pointing at Merv) want all the cookies!" Merv smiles and munches his cookie. He has no intention of giving away even one of them.

Sharon's simple interpretation of Merv's message and her cheerful acceptance of the slice of cheese clearly reflect Merv's intent, as well as communicating her appreciation of his sense of humour. Merv learns a great deal from this interaction.

One of the many benefits of interpreting your partner's message is that this can become a catalyst for speech if your partner has the potential to talk. Part 2 of Polly and Shawn's story from page 35 illustrates this principle:

In response to Polly's requests, Shawn has inserted the cassette into the tape recorder, but Polly still has to solve the problem of power — the tape recorder is unplugged. Once again, Shawn waits for Polly to communicate as he watches her struggle to insert the plug into the socket. Finally, she stands up and gives Shawn the cord. He interprets, "Help please", and is unexpectedly rewarded when Polly imitates him and says, "Hep peese". This is the first time he has heard her imitate speech in a meaningful way.

By holding back and waiting for Polly to initiate, Shawn has discovered that Polly is quite capable of communicating intentionally with gestures. However, when he **interprets her message at her level**, he finds out that she can imitate spoken language and use it meaningfully! Polly is still a long way from speaking consistently, but Shawn now knows that, with opportunity and appropriate language models, she can learn.

Interpreting your partner's message is a very important part of communicating with her, but this can be challenging:

- when her understanding of speech is limited
- when you can't figure out what she is trying to tell you; and
- when her messages are neither intentional nor consistent

There are specific ways to approach each of these situations . . .

How to interpret when your partner's understanding of speech is limited . . .

When your partner's ability to understand speech is limited, you need to make your interpretation of her message clear **by using your body when you talk**.

Using your body when you interpret your partner's messages makes it much easier for her to understand the connection between her message and yours. Actions and gestures not only attract and hold your partner's interest, but they make learning easier and more fun. They validate the way she communicates at the same time as they provide a model for how *she* can use *her* body to communicate with you.

Partners who communicate at Levels 1, 2 or 3 will benefit most from having their messages interpreted using actions and gestures that are clear and recognizable. However, even partners who communicate at Level 4 will benefit from your use of clear body language.

When using body language, you can:

- **Point** — to what you think your partner is talking about
- **Gesture** — what your partner seems to be telling you
- **Show** — the item or action your partner seems to be talking about
- **Use facial expressions** — to let your face register the emotion your partner seems to be expressing

When your partner lets you know that:

she	you interpret by saying	and you use your body to add meaning by
is hungry	"Hungry. You're hungry."	patting your stomach
is tired	"Tired? Go to sleep."	placing your head on your hand and closing your eyes

Interpret your partner's messages with a combination of words and gestures.

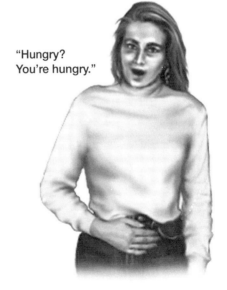

"Hungry? You're hungry."

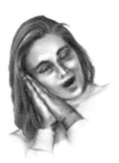

"Tired? Go to sleep."

Interpret your partner's messages with a combination of words and gestures.

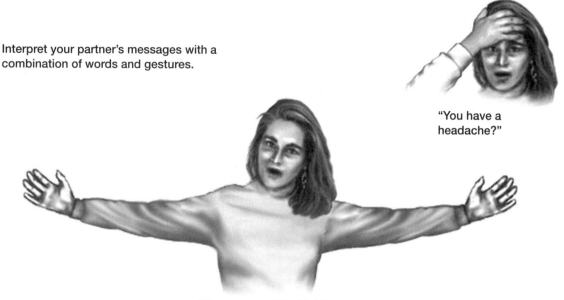

"You have a headache?"

"The van was **this** big?"

she	you interpret by saying	and you use your body to add meaning by
has a headache	"You have a headache?"	holding your hand on your forehead and grimacing
saw a **very** big van	"The van was this big?"	holding your arms out on either side of you as you say "this big"

How to interpret when you can't understand what your partner is trying to tell you . . .

The best thing to do when you can't understand your partner is to make an educated guess at what she is trying to say. She will be the first to let you know if, in some way, you've misinterpreted. If she communicates at or beyond Level 3, she will let you know directly that you have misinterpreted. If her communication is not sophisticated enough to do this, it may take some time before you realize that the two of you are not communicating about the same thing.

In the following examples, let's assume that all of your partner's messages are unclear and that your interpretations are missing the mark:

Nancy communicates at Level 1:

NANCY: Smiles when you come in with some food.
YOU: Smile. *"Oh, **food**! You want to **eat**!"*

Nancy may not have been hungry at all. You find this out when you try to give her something to eat, and she clamps her mouth shut. If you have to make a guess at why she smiled, you might end up thinking that she was just pleased to see you!

Tony communicates at Level 2:

TONY: Begins to reach toward a book on the table.

YOU: Point to the book. *"Book? You want the **book**?"*

Tony may not be interested in the book. On the other side of the book, there is a cassette tape that he wants. The trick now is for you to figure out if he wants to have the music played, or if he simply wants to tap the cassette on the table.

Mike communicates at Level 3:

MIKE: Pulls you toward an arcade section of the mall and points. *"Pay!"*

YOU: *"**Play**! You want to **play** a **game**?"*

Thinking that Mike wants to play a video game, you walk with him to the arcade and head for the games section. But Mike drags you away from the games, repeating, "Pay! Pay!" You interpret, "You don't want to play here. You want to go somewhere else." He pulls you towards another section of the arcade where there is an antique piano that he has obviously seen before. *This* is what he wants to play.

Linda and Kelly both communicate at Level 4:

LINDA: Gestures the action of pulling teeth. *"Teef!"*

YOU: *"Teeth. Your dentist pulled your teeth?"*

Linda responds to your interpretation with a firm "No!" She gives you more information: "Wauf!" You repeat: "Wauf?" Eventually you remember that she has a nephew named Ralph. You interpret, "Ralph! Ralph had a tooth pulled!" She grins and nods. You finally got it right.

KELLY: (picture board user) Stretches for a cup on the table which is out of reach.

YOU: Point to the picture of "want" and "coffee". *"Kelly, you want coffee."*

The smile on Kelly's face fades when you interpret "Kelly, you want coffee". You start narrowing down the choices. You try "Tea?", but she continues to look at you. What else could be hot? "Milk?" No luck. "Water?" Her face lights up. (Well, some people like hot water!)

Amos communicates at Level 5:

AMOS (who is verbal):	*"Ahwe mawbie."*
YOU:	*You went to a movie?*

Amos tries again, but you still don't understand him. He says, "No" and drags you to the living room where he picks up a book. He was trying to tell you: "I went to the library."

From time to time, you may be unable to figure out what your partner is trying to say and, eventually, you will have to tell her so. While she may become frustrated, your sincere effort to interpret her message will confirm for her that communicating is still worthwhile, even though this time it was not successful. Sometimes it is the simple act of interacting, rather than being understood, that is rewarding to your partner.

How to interpret when your partner's messages are neither intentional nor consistent . . .

The only way your partner will learn that her actions and sounds have the power to communicate is by seeing them interpreted.

If your partner randomly touches an object, interpret this as a request or as an attempt to show you something. Respond either by labelling the object and giving it to her or by showing her what it is used for. Allow her a choice between objects, and give her the first thing she reaches for. In time, her actions and sounds will acquire meaning in her mind because they elicit a predictable response from you.

Follow your partner's lead: IMITATE what your partner says and does

Imitating your partner helps you connect with her at a level that she can understand.

You can imitate your partner's:

- actions
- sounds
- signs
- words
- facial expressions

When you follow your partner's lead by imitating her, she experiences a sense of empowerment that motivates her to keep the interaction going. The results can be truly amazing. By imitating, you can establish a rapport with someone very quickly, even if you have just met! You can capture your partner's attention and give her behaviour new meaning. And you become more sensitive to her interests and to her messages.

Imitating the actions of partners who communicate at Level 2 can help you make a connection which might not otherwise be made. . .

Mary, who is confined to a wheelchair, communicates non-verbally at Level 2. Her facilitator, Frank, knows that she likes activities that involve her senses. He sprays shaving cream onto her tray and gently places her hand in the cream. She smiles and so does he, as he says "Shaving cream". Then, as he dots her nose with cream, he says "On your nose." She looks at him, he looks at her, and they smile at each other. He then says "On your hand", and rubs shaving cream on her hand. He pauses, with her hand still underneath his. They look at each other again, and then slowly and tentatively, Mary moves her hand out from under Frank's hand and places it on top of his hand. Frank, realizing that she might be onto a new game, imitates her, removing his hand from under hers and placing it on top of her hand. Before long they are involved in a game of slapping hands, made all the more interesting by the sound and feel of the shaving cream sealing and releasing.

Imitation works wonders with partners who communicate at Level 3 . . .

Toni is a Level 3 communicator. At work, she constantly takes her shoes and socks off, and her facilitators constantly tell her to put them back on. Jill, one of her facilitators, decides to try something different. She decides to follow Toni's lead — maybe she can use imitation to turn this activity into an interactive game.

*With both of them on the floor, Toni takes her shoes off one by one. So Jill imitates her and takes **her** shoes off one by one. Toni sees this and pauses; this isn't part of the regular routine! Unexpectedly, she reaches for one of Jill's shoes and slips it onto her own foot. Jill smiles and waits to see what Toni will do next. Toni picks up one of her own shoes and hands it to Jill, who slips it on (even though it is too small!). Toni then takes Jill's shoe off and slips off her sock. Jill imitates her and slips her sock off too. Toni pauses, then puts her sock back on again, and so does Jill.*

By imitating Toni's actions, Jill engages her in an activity for up to 20 minutes before she calls it quits. This also gives Jill plenty of opportunities to model the signs for "sock" and "shoe" and gestures for "you", "me" and "pull".

Imitating your partner who communicates at Level 4 can be a lot of fun . . .

Beth-Anne is a small woman who has Down Syndrome and who communicates at Level 4. Beth-Anne really enjoys counting. She and Ellen, her facilitator, are sitting together in front of a box of craft materials; Ellen's plan is to make a small flower. Suddenly Beth-Anne stands up, begins pumping her arms and counting "One! Two! Fee!" Ellen also stands up, pumps her arms, and counts "One! Two! Three!" Beth-Anne continues, this time pumping even harder. Ellen follows suit, and the interaction continues until they both get so tired, they collapse, panting and laughing together.

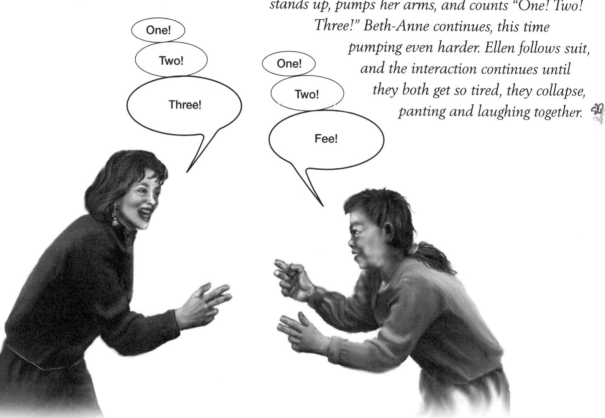

Ellen abandons the craft activity and imitates Beth-Anne's counting, which leads to an interaction that is more fun for them both.

As a result of Ellen's willingness to participate in Beth-Anne's chosen activity at a moment's notice, Beth-Anne enjoys the interaction immensely and will soon be ready to learn more sophisticated communication skills from Ellen.

Imitate — but provide a correct model

People who are at the early stages of language development often mispronounce words or use incorrect grammar and vocabulary. If your partners are to develop more mature ways of expressing themselves, they need to hear how their message sounds when it is said *correctly*. This is called **modelling**.

When your partner:	You can:
Mispronounces words: e.g., "tedda" for sweater	**Model the correct pronunciation:** "Sweater"
Uses immature grammar: e.g., "Wanna see movie"	**Model a complete sentence:** "You want to see a movie."
Uses incorrect signs: e.g. "cheese" by clapping hands together	**Interpret with words and model the correct sign:** e.g., Say "cheese" while pressing palms together and twisting, which is the correct symbol for "cheese".
Uses incorrect labels: e.g., "meat" while reaching for cheese	**Model the correct word:** Point to cheese and say "Cheese"

When you interpret, imitate or model for your partner, she obtains the information she needs to improve. Best of all, the conversation is not interrupted as it would be if you stopped to tell her that she has made an error.

LET'S REVIEW

You play many roles with your partner, and these roles can affect how well your partner interacts and communicates with you.

You can play:

- the "Helper"
- the "Mover"
- the "Director"

All these roles can help your partners learn something — if they aren't overused. Yet the best conversational partner is the **"Responsive Conversation Partner"**.

As a "Responsive Conversation Partner", you stop focusing on what *you* expect from *your partner* and focus on what your partner is telling you. You give her the opportunity to express what is on her mind by **allowing her to lead**. You follow her lead, **responding immediately** to her messages, **interpreting** or **imitating** them and **providing correct models** for spoken messages.

As a "Responsive Conversation Partner", you "go with the flow", letting your partner take the initiative and communicate about what interests her. As a result, your partner learns to be confident that what she says or does will receive the type of response she is looking for.

As a "Responsive Conversation Partner", you **use your body** both when you interpret your partner's messages and during everyday communication. You use the same communicative actions your partner uses, such as pointing, gesturing and various facial expressions. These movements, while making the meaning clearer, also add animation and interest, as well as modelling new ways for your partner to communicate.

When it is hard to understand what your partner is trying to say, remember that "Responsive Conversation Partners" try to make educated guesses or try again later.

If you're having a hard time encouraging your partner to participate in a conversation, it could be because of her conversational style, which might be:

- a person with her own agenda
- reluctant
- passive
- sociable

Your partner may demonstrate any of these styles, depending on the situation and her comfort with it. As her partner, you must be alert to these styles so that you can **adapt** your behaviour to encourage your partner to lead and initiate. (More on this in the next chapter!)

Chapter Three Adapt Activities So You and Your Partner Can Share Them

"Where opportunity doesn't knock, build a door." **MILTON BERLE**

To a large extent, the quality of our lives depends on how well we are integrated into our communities. The more involved we are in community activities, the more connected we feel to others and the more fulfilling life becomes.

In order for your partners to feel like members of their communities, they also need to participate in the world around them. Unfortunately, many people who are developmentally delayed do not participate in a variety of routines and activities — not because they aren't capable, but because they are *perceived* as not being capable.

Because many of your partners have limited speech or none at all, they may not be *expected* to communicate or participate in activities. When participation is not expected, it is not offered. As a result, your partners may find themselves left out of those incidental, everyday interactions which most people take for granted. When this happens, your partners learn that their full contribution to the activities, events and relationships in their lives is not expected or required. Sometimes it is even denied.

The solution to this problem is not a complicated one. It involves making adaptations that enable your partners to experience full participation in their communities. This is a grand vision which can be achieved through the sharing of simple, everyday activities and interests.

When you share activities with your partner, genuine conversations will occur. Your responsiveness and willingness to share yourself let him know that he is worthy of your attention. When you create special times together, you encourage him to become a more active communicator. Adapting activities so they can be shared will enable your partner to use his existing communication skills more often, as well as to learn new ones.

This chapter is about what you can do to create shared experiences that will open your partner to learning. In this chapter, you will:

- learn to adapt daily activities and routines so you can share them with your partner

- learn to adapt leisure activities so that your partner can partici-pate with you at his own level

- To make every shared activity the "right" kind of activity, you will need to:

Base these activities on your partner's preferred interest patterns and on his daily living activities — to ensure that there are built-in opportunities for both of you to participate and communicate

Know your partner's level of communication — so you can be realistic about the kind of communication you can expect from him

Allow your partner to lead — and respond immediately to his messages

SHARE DAILY ACTIVITIES AND ROUTINES

It is within the rhythms and motions of everyday life that you and your partner have the most contact. From sunup to sundown you have opportunities to share activities and events. You prepare and eat meals together; you help your partner perform everyday routines such as dressing and grooming; you shop and do laundry together. It is within such mundane, routine activities that friendship and trust are built, especially if your focus is on interaction, rather than on completion of the task.

Get involved in the activity yourself!

Instead of watching and instructing your partner through daily routines — get involved yourself!

Zina is non-verbal and communicates intentionally (although infrequently) at Level 3. Every day, she makes her own lunch. Her facilitator, Jacob, usually sits and watches her, prompting her at each step. Zina frequently interrupts this activity to engage in self-stimulation, looking at the ceiling and shaking the object in her hand. She rarely communicates when she makes her lunch.

Today, Zina is making herself a sandwich. Jacob decides to adapt the activity by joining in and making himself a sandwich at the same time. Surprised, Zina stops self-stimulating and watches him intently. After a few minutes, she unexpectedly dips her knife into the bottle of cheese spread and then extends it toward him. She seems to want help with the cheese spread. *Stay tuned . . . the story continues on page 51 . . .*

Do something different, unusual or unexpected to encourage interaction

Sometimes sharing an activity may not result in improved interaction. You and your partner may find yourselves doing the same thing alongside one another, without any communication or interaction. In this case, you need to do more.

You may need to attract your partner's attention by doing something unusual or unexpected — something that obliges him to participate and communicate.

There are many ways to build in opportunities for your partner to communicate during daily activities:

- don't provide a needed item
- limit the number of items provided so they have to be shared
- dispense items to your partner one at a time and wait for him to request another
- place familiar items in a new spot
- place necessary items out of reach, though within view
- reorganize familiar areas
- discreetly unplug small, commonly used appliances
- innocently hand your partner an item that will not work in the activity — e.g., a slotted spoon to serve soup
- respond too literally to your partner's communications
- respond to your partner in a way he does not expect

Because your goal is to encourage successful interaction and to avoid confusion or frustration, you must ensure that your partner is familiar with a routine before you change or adapt it. If you don't, he won't recognize that you are doing something different and won't be able to respond appropriately.

Adaptations of routines can occur in different forms and at different stages of the routine. For example, before setting the table one day, you might put the cutlery tray, which is normally on the counter, out of reach but within view. If your partner responds by pointing this out to you or by requesting in some way that you give him the cutlery, the next day you might repeat this. Then you could revert to having the cutlery tray within reach, but after a few days you might put only spoons in it.

Initially, when you do something unexpected during a familiar routine, your partner may look surprised and may not respond immediately. **Wait** and look expectant, giving him as much time as he needs to communicate. Soon enough he *will* respond, and interaction will become an established part of the routine.

The important part about adapting routines is to pace the changes, to use them every now and again as a way to increase communication. They should not be overused.

Diane, who is at Level 2, rarely communicates with Michelle, her facilitator. One of Diane's favourite activities is folding towels. Normally, Michelle takes a whole load of towels from the dryer and places them in a basket for Diane to fold. This time, Michelle adapts the routine and gives Diane one towel at a time.

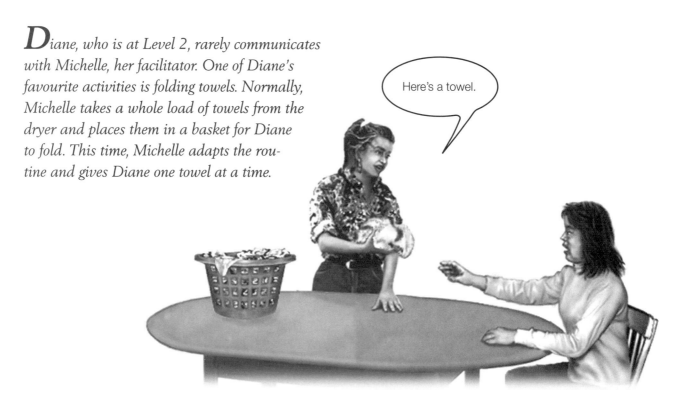

Michelle hands Diane a towel to fold.

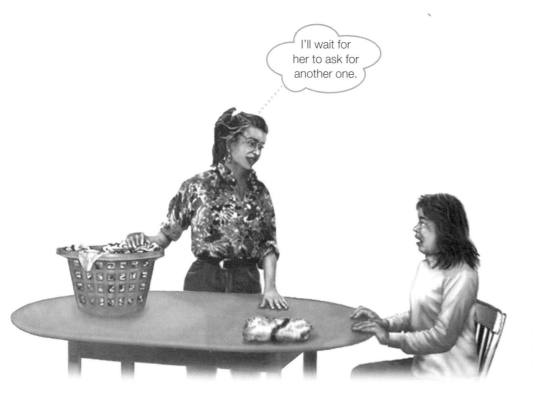

Once the towel has been folded, Michelle waits for Diane to let her know that she wants another one.

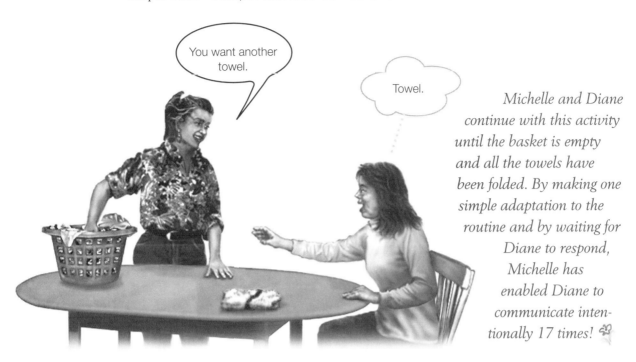

Michelle and Diane continue with this activity until the basket is empty and all the towels have been folded. By making one simple adaptation to the routine and by waiting for Diane to respond, Michelle has enabled Diane to communicate intentionally 17 times! 🌿

Michelle's waiting pays off — Diane reaches for another towel.

Let's look at another example of an adapted routine as Zina's story continues from page 48. Not only does Zina (a Level 3 communicator) learn about the power of communication from her interaction with Jacob, but she also discovers the consequences of sending an unclear message.

Zina is holding out her knife to Jacob because she wants him to spread the cheese onto her bread for her . . . 🌿

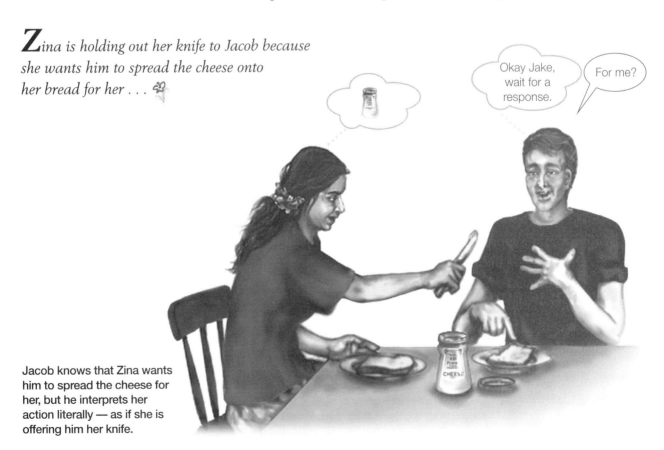

Jacob knows that Zina wants him to spread the cheese for her, but he interprets her action literally — as if she is offering him her knife.

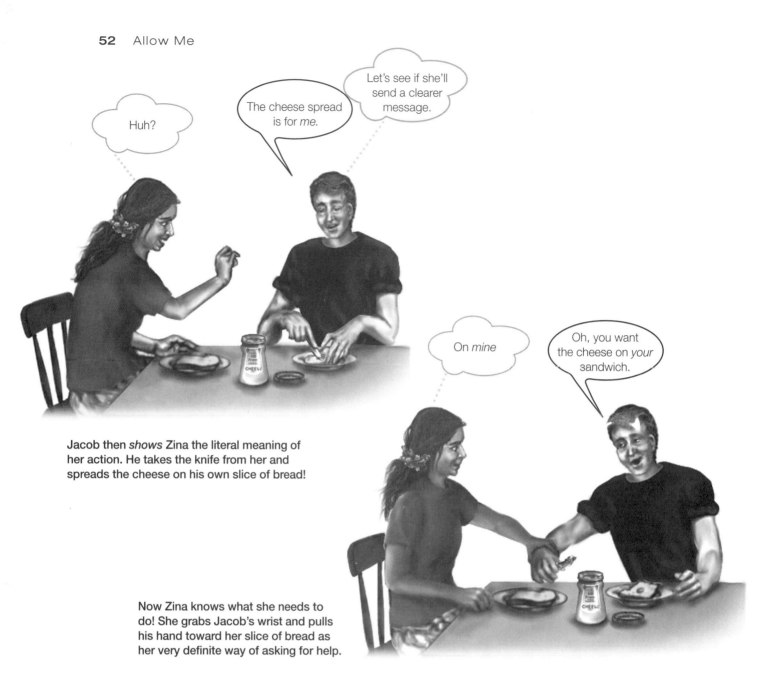

Jacob then *shows* Zina the literal meaning of her action. He takes the knife from her and spreads the cheese on his own slice of bread!

Now Zina knows what she needs to do! She grabs Jacob's wrist and pulls his hand toward her slice of bread as her very definite way of asking for help.

Novelty and surprise will help Zina learn to communicate for a variety of purposes. In this story, she communicates to make a request. In other situations, she may communicate to refuse, to direct her facilitator's actions or to point out mistakes. She needs to communicate in many different situations in order to become a more versatile communicator.

REMEMBER . . . For your partner to learn flexible ways of communicating, you need to build some flexibility and change into the way activities and routines are conducted.

The most important thing is to use adaptations gently, wisely and sensitively so as to maintain your partner's trust while you encourage him to learn from you.

SHARE LEISURE AND RECREATIONAL ACTIVITIES

Leisure and recreational activities are an important part of our lives. These activities include social activities (such as going to dances, local pubs and to people's homes), physical activities (like skiing, skating or golfing), as well as more intellectual activities (like classical music concerts, museums and the theatre).

Most of us have an enormous range of leisure activities from which to choose. However, the range of leisure activities available to people with developmental delays may be extremely limited. Because independence is generally considered to be a priority for this group of people, it is possible that their leisure skills have been sacrificed to the acquisition of self-help and motor skills. As a result, your partners may have had few opportunities to learn how to play or they may have lost the play skills they once had.

Curiously, people with developmental delays behave very differently when they go camping during the summer. They are more communicative, more enthusiastic, friendlier and happier. What does this tell us about them, about their ability to be amused, to interact, to learn new skills? It tells us that, like everyone else, they need variety and laughter in their lives.

As a "Responsive Conversation Partner", you can offer your partner opportunities for playfulness and fun that will encourage interaction which, in turn, will promote communication. So, let's start by focusing on what your partner enjoys doing. In Chapter 1, you determined your partner's patterns of interest. Look back at his preferred activities and see if you can share these in any way. How could you adapt these to heighten his participation and enjoyment? Are there common themes among his favourite activities which give you some ideas for introducing new activities?

Identifying a number of pleasurable activities that you and your partner can share is the critical first step. When your partner is motivated to participate in shared activities, there's no limit to what he can gain from these positive, enjoyable interactions.

Adapt activities that involve early sensory experiences

Spending time with a partner who is deeply focused on sensory stimulation can be difficult because such a partner rarely initiates social contact. Therefore, the onus is on *you* to engage him so he can learn to interact with others.

Join in your partner's solitary activity by **following his lead and imitating what he does**. He will become aware of you when you relate to him at his level. Tap objects on a table with him, rock your body as he rocks his, flip through magazines together. This is an unstressful time in which you place few or no demands on him. Your goal is to promote his awareness of others which, in time, can lead to the development of intentional communication.

Jerry is considered to be a reflexive communicator (Level 1). Confined to a wheelchair, he enjoys rocking and engages in little else. His facilitator, Irene, decides to spend some time with him while he is out of his wheelchair, seated on the gym floor. Jerry, as expected, begins to rock. Irene, who has seated herself on the floor opposite him, imitates his rocking, then waits. To her surprise, Jerry slowly moves closer to her every time he rocks. Irene imitates him by moving closer to him too. He finally stops as their noses touch. For several seconds, he looks into her eyes. Then slowly he rocks away again. Jerry's new game continues for up to half an hour, until Irene decides to call it quits. She is so excited — this is the first time he has demonstrated an awareness of anyone.

Irene's sharing of this activity on Jerry's terms has motivated him to communicate and, to her surprise, to employ some Level 2 behaviours. As Jerry became *aware* of Irene, he included her in his world by looking at her, moving closer to her and by imitating her. His movements and pauses, unintentional at first, became more deliberate and the activity became a **shared** sensory activity.

Adapt leisure routines

There are two ways to approach sharing leisure routines with your partner, both of which will increase the **frequency** of his communication:

- **Use a familiar routine and introduce something new or unexpected**

  The principles that apply to adapting daily routines apply equally to adapting leisure routines. First, find a way of participating in the routine with your partner. Then introduce something new or unexpected, while maintaining the structure of the rest of the routine.

- **Introduce a new leisure routine**

  Keep trying new routines that are consistent with your partner's interests. Your awareness of your partner's likes and preferences will help you become creative in your efforts to expand his repertoire of leisure activities.

Remember, however, that when your partner is learning a new routine, he must know it well before you introduce any changes or adaptations to it. Once you introduce a change to the routine, your judicious use of **waiting** will be the key to encouraging him to communicate with you.

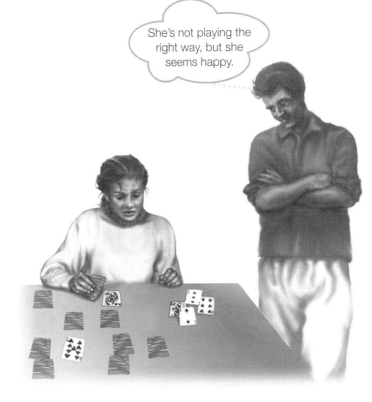

*V*era, a Level 4 communicator, loves to play with Memory cards. She does this almost daily, making up her own rules. Russ, her facilitator, has never joined in her game.

Vera's version of Memory involves turning over two cards and putting them in a "pairs" pile, whether they match or not. As usual, Russ stands and watches.

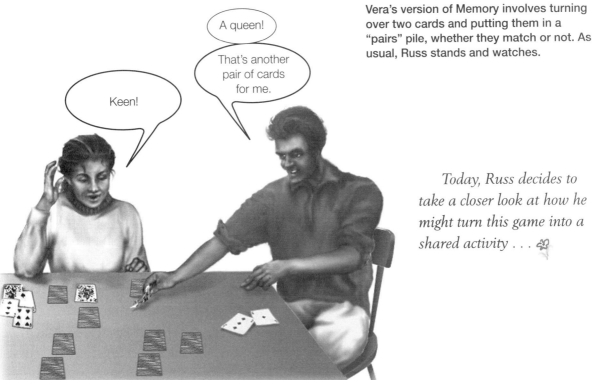

Today, Russ decides to take a closer look at how he might turn this game into a shared activity . . .

When Russ joins in and plays Memory, Vera gets excited, naming the cards as a way of interacting with him. Russ then provides a correct model, which not only helps Vera learn to express herself better, but makes the game more fun for both of them.

Adapt creative activities

People approach creative activities in a variety of ways. Some create in conventional ways, while others prefer to "do their own thing". Your partner may have his own way of approaching a creative activity, and his way might be quite different from yours. If your partner wants to do the activity one way and you another, a potentially enjoyable activity can become frustrating and painful. If you are to share his activity, you need to abandon your own agenda and beliefs about the "right" way to approach the activity.

Keep the creative juices flowing when you share the activity:

- allow your partner to "do his own thing"
- imitate — do what he does or do something similar
- slowly introduce new ways of being creative at his level

*H*olly *communicates at Level 3, using gestures. She is shy and slow to communicate. She has access to a picture communication book, but she does not appear to know what it is for.*

Holly enjoys putting simple items together from kits. She either does this by herself or with her facilitators watching her and she always ignores their frequent admonitions to put the pieces together according to the kit's instructions.

Holly has a new owl kit to assemble, and Jean, one of her facilitators, wants to do it with her. Jean makes a conscious effort to let Holly direct the activity and watches closely to see what Holly will do. Holly begins to apply glue to pieces of pre-cut felt, so Jean asks if she can help. Holly smiles and gives her some felt pieces and, for a while, they both apply glue to the felt pieces. When this is done, Jean waits for Holly to direct the next stage. Holly gives Jean a piece of felt and points to the spot where she wants Jean to put it. Jean follows Holly's instructions to the letter. Although the kit is designed to produce an owl, they have produced their own eclectic piece of artwork, and Holly is beaming. ❧

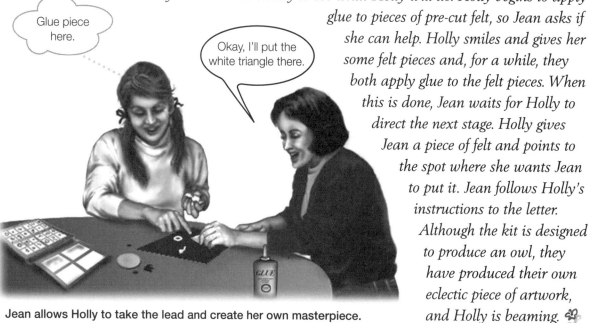

Jean allows Holly to take the lead and create her own masterpiece.

After sharing her artwork in this way a few times, Holly is always eager to interact with Jean. By allowing Holly to lead, Jean has come to know how Holly likes to create, which makes the time they spend together more enjoyable and very much more interactive. Soon it will be Holly's turn to join in one of Jean's creative activities. While they create works of art together, they are building a genuine relationship.

REMEMBER . . . Shared activities are the foundation on which conversational and communication skills are built. Without being together — without sharing — there would be no reason to communicate. Your partner's desire to interact with others in enjoyable, shared activities will motivate him to tune in and to learn.

LET'S REVIEW

You encourage your partner to participate in the rhythms of life when you:

Adapt daily routines to share them with your partner:

- get involved in your partner's daily routines and activities
- design routines and activities to give your partner more opportunities to participate
- do something new, unusual or unexpected to encourage your partner to communicate

Create opportunities for playfulness and interaction during recreational and leisure activities:

- determine your partner's pattern of interests (sensory, leisure, creative)
- share activities that are of interest to your partner, allowing him to lead
- introduce new activities that share the characteristics of those your partner prefers
- ensure your partner is familiar with these routines
- change and adapt familiar routines to encourage interaction

Chapter Four Get the Conversation Going and Keep It Going

Conversation allows people to do many things: to participate in activities, to learn, to share experiences, to get to know others and to express who they are. Conversation is a give-and-take affair, with each conversation partner having to contribute and participate. In order to have successful, enjoyable conversations, both partners must know the rules of conversation — and there are many! The most basic rules include: taking and giving a turn when appropriate; building on what was said in the previous turn; and repeating or clarifying what was said when the listener looks confused or responds inappropriately.

It can be very difficult to hold a conversation with a partner if she doesn't know the basic rules of conversation and if her language skills are limited. When we find it difficult to communicate with someone, the conversation tends to be short, one-sided and not very enjoyable for either party. The only way your partner can improve her conversational skills is to have frequent conversations with an experienced, skillful partner — like you. As the more competent conversationalist, your task is to structure the conversation so that she can keep taking turns. You have to ensure that your turn keeps her engaged and makes it relatively easy for her to take the next turn. In this way, you support her participation in extended conversations.

There are many benefits to your partner's regular and ongoing participation in extended conversations, the main ones being that she develops increased self-confidence, learns a great deal about the world and discovers how communication is used to maintain social interaction.

In this chapter, you will learn:

- what a conversation consists of

- how partners at different levels of communication can take turns in a conversation

- how to get a conversation going with your partner

- how to keep the conversation going using appropriate questions and signals

WHAT IS A CONVERSATION?

A conversation is an exchange of information between people and is made up of a series of turns.

For example:

SUE: Have you heard about Anne? (opening turn, which is a question)

JOHN: No, what about her? (turn is a response to the question, followed by another question)

SUE: She's leaving her job and going to travel the world. (turn provides information requested)

JOHN: What made her decide to do that? (turn requests additional information)

SUE: Well, she says she's always wanted to travel and the longer she waits, the less likely she is to do it. (turn provides requested information)

JOHN: She's probably right. I'd love to do that one day. (turn provides information)

SUE: So would I — maybe some day, when I win the lottery. Well, I'd better get back to work. See you later. (turn provides information, signals the end of the conversation)

JOHN: Yes, bye. (turn ends conversation)

In conversations, we exchange information about each other's lives, activities, interests and opinions. In genuine conversations, people learn a lot about each other that they did not know before, especially if the conversation continues for several turns.

Most people think of conversations as involving speech. However, a turn in a conversation can be verbal or non-verbal. All of us have had the experience of saying something during a conversation and seeing our listener respond with an offended or surprised look. Non-verbal behaviours like these send us important messages, and we treat them as a turn. We respond to the emotion or intention of the nonverbal information, even if the spoken words send a different message.

Anything that sends a message to another person is a turn. When you talk to your partner, she may take her turn using a gesture, a look, a change in facial expression, a sound or words. As long as you are both focused on the same topic and you continue to take turns, you are having a conversation.

There are many ways to take a turn . . .

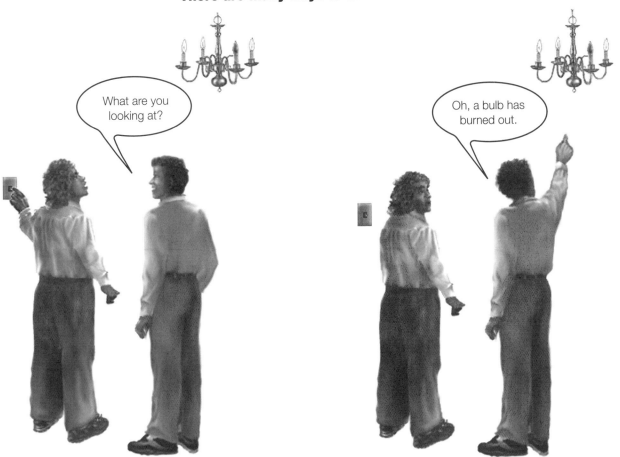

This person took a turn by pointing.

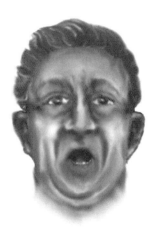

This person took his turn by changing his facial expression.

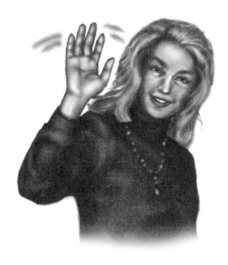

This person took her turn by using a gesture.

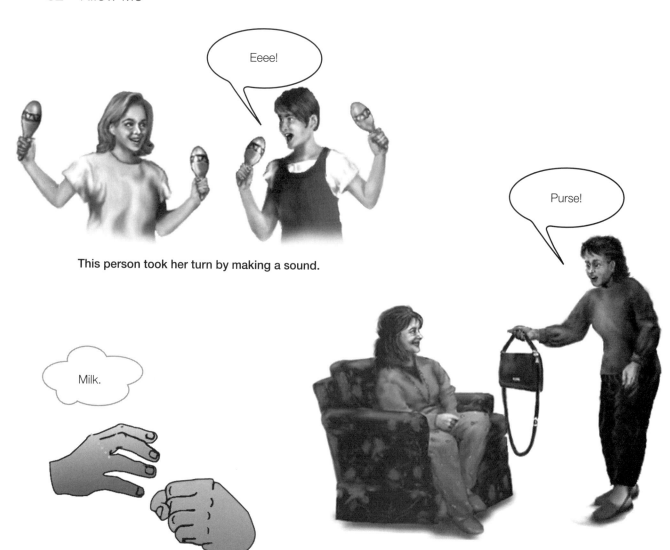

This person took her turn by making a sound.

This person took her turn by saying a word.

This turn involves making a sign.

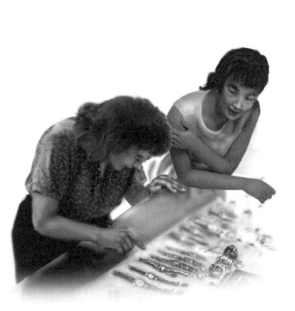

This person took her turn by pointing to an object.

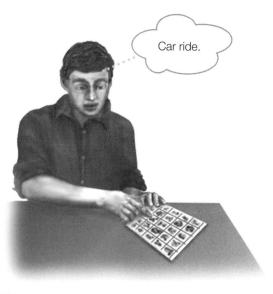

This person took his turn by pointing to a picture.

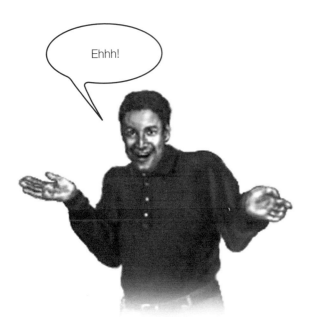

This person took his turn by combining actions and sounds.

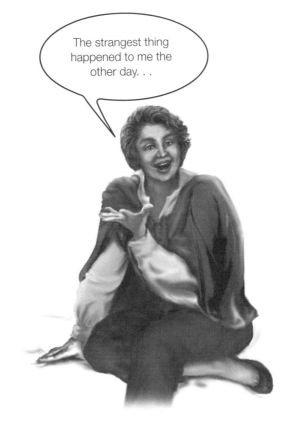

This person took her turn by speaking.

Being a competent conversation partner means being able to *initiate* conversations as well as being able to respond when others initiate them. It's important for your partner to be given opportunities to participate in conversations that she initiates as well as in those initiated by others.

In the following examples, first the facilitator initiates the conversation and then his partner does.

Jim, a facilitator, and his partner, Matthew, are standing at the window, looking at snow falling. Jim initiates:

JIM: (facilitator):   *"Look at the snow outside!"*
MATTHEW: Looks at snow; touches the window pane.
JIM: *"It looks cold!"* Shivers.
MATTHEW: *"Hoho."*
JIM: *"Yes, it's like Christmas! It looks like Christmas outside!"*
MATTHEW: Goes to closet and gets his boots.
JIM: *"You've got your boots! You want to go outside in the snow!"*

Later, Jim and Matthew are outside in the snow, and Matthew initiates:

MATTHEW (partner): Crouches in the snow and begins to roll a large snowball. Turns to look at Jim.

JIM: Watches Matthew, smiling.

MATTHEW: Tugs at Jim with one hand, points to his snowball on the ground with the other and grunts. *"Uh! Uh!"*

JIM: *"Oh, you want me to roll a snowball too. Okay."*

MATTHEW: After the snowballs are made, he pats one and points to the other while looking at Jim.

JIM: *"A snowman! You want to build a snowman!"*

MATTHEW: Signs. *"Yes."*

JIM: *"Okay, let's put your snowball on top of mine. We'll make a snowman."*

SET UP CONVERSATIONS FOR SUCCESS

Not all conversations help our partners express themselves, especially if they are one-sided. When one person takes all the turns in a conversation, the other person has no opportunity to participate, learn, share and achieve. It is as if she were on a seesaw with her feet dangling in the air while the other person's feet are firmly planted on the ground. For conversations to be positive, they have to be balanced, with both partners participating equally. Even if your partner is unable to speak, she can and should be given the opportunity to take an equal number of turns.

There are a number of tools at your disposal to get and keep the conversation going with your partner, all of which can be used naturally during the course of the conversation.

GET the conversation going

In order to *get* the conversation going, you can use the usual conversational openers such as questions, comments, teasing and roughhousing. However, it is important to encourage your partner to *initiate* the conversation by setting the stage for her to communicate.

The following two strategies will encourage your partner to **begin** the conversation:

- be face-to-face
- wait, observe and listen

GET the conversation going: Be face-to-face

Being face-to-face is a vital part of encouraging someone to communicate with you. When you look directly into your partner's eyes, it communicates your interest and encourages her to initiate. In addition, she can watch your facial expressions, gestures and words and can become better able to understand your emotions and intents. This is especially true for partners in wheelchairs. Being face-to-face also enables you to recognize and respond to your partner's subtle efforts to communicate. Once you are face-to-face, try to stay that way — it will encourage your partner to keep interacting with you.

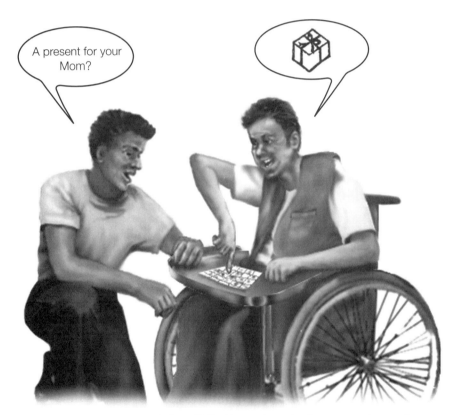

Partners in wheelchairs will find it much easier to communicate when they are face-to-face with you.

GET the conversation going: Wait, observe and listen

The best conversationalists tend to be the best listeners. We all enjoy talking to someone who is genuinely interested in what we have to say and who listens, without interrupting us or looking away. The same principle applies to people with limited abilities to communicate — they communicate more readily and remain engaged for longer with people who give them a chance to communicate and then listen well.

KEEP the conversation going

Your partner's ability to keep the conversation going is affected by a number of things. If she is interested in what's being discussed or in the ongoing activity, she'll stay involved longer. A good attention span helps her to stay focused, even when she's less enthusiastic about the topic of the conversation. However, your skill as a conversation partner can significantly affect how long she stays with you and continues taking turns. For example, the longer you stay on topic, giving her ample time and opportunity to respond, the more likely she is to contribute to the conversation — and the more she will learn. In addition, when you take *your* turn in such a way that you set her up to succeed in taking *hers*, she may demonstrate conversational skills you never knew she had.

To **keep** the conversation going:

- show your pleasure and interest
- use questions that continue the conversation and limit those that don't
- use signals to encourage your partner to take another turn

KEEP the conversation going: Show your pleasure and interest

What really matters in a conversation is your sincere desire to connect with your conversation partner. This comes through in many ways, and you can't fake it! Smiling is an obvious way to show this, but other body language works too. When your eyes are wide open and you lean forward and look expectant, you communicate your interest in having a conversation. Your delight in "sharing the moment" with your partner will stimulate her interest and create the fertile ground in which learning can grow.

You can:

Look at your partner — there's nothing like good eye contact to make your partner feel important.

Smile or laugh — everyone enjoys the company of someone who is fun to be around.

Move close to your partner — it is hard for her to ignore you when you are physically close to her; but don't get so close that her personal space is violated.

Exaggerate your facial expressions — raise your eyebrows and act surprised if your partner expresses something unusual.

Use energy in your voice and movements — animation will capture and maintain your partner's interest.

Lean forward — to show your partner she has your focus and interest.

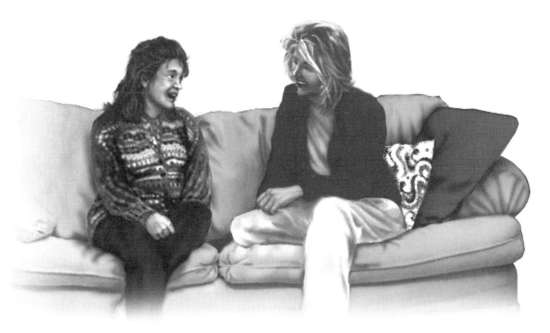

Being close to your partner creates an atmosphere of warmth and reduces outside distractions.

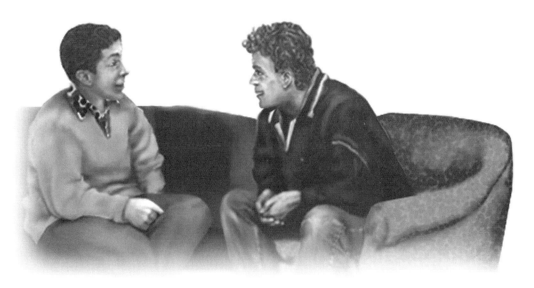

Lean forward to show your interest.

KEEP the conversation going: Use questions that continue the conversation and limit those that don't

Questions are a necessary part of every conversation, and when used well, they allow the conversation to flow. But when they are misused, questions can bring conversations to a grinding halt. Many of us have tried to keep conversations going with our partners by asking question after question, only to get no response at all. Although this overuse of questions reflects our natural response to a conversation partner who is hard to engage, it seldom works. In fact, it can backfire, making our partner communicate even less!

Your questions may discourage your partner from taking another turn if they:

- **test, bombard or demand responses** — e.g., "What do you call that?" "What do you use a knife for?"
- **are rhetorical** — e.g., "You don't want milk, do you? "
- **are too difficult for your partner to understand** — e.g., "Why do you think she didn't call at the usual time?"
- **limit your partner's response** — e.g., by asking for a "yes" or "no" answer when your partner is able to give more complete answers
- **are used indirectly to control behaviour** — e.g., "Do you want to clear the table now?"

Questions that keep the conversation going:

- are genuine and appropriate
- are clearly related to the topic of the conversation
- are focused on what your partner is interested in
- are used to check that you have understood your partner's message
- are used to get information that you need or are interested in
- are geared to your partner's ability to understand and communicate

REMEMBER . . . The right kind of question is one which helps your partner take another turn — not just any turn — but one which enables her to draw upon her communication skills and to stay on topic.

Adjust your questions to your partner's communication level

When used well, questions are geared to a partner's ability to understand language and to express herself. Questions that can be answered with actions or with one-word answers are appropriate for partners at the early stages of language and communication development. But these kinds of questions may be limiting if overused with a partner who is able to speak in short sentences or to combine words using signs or other symbols.

For example, if your partner can only identify an object by pointing, then an appropriate question is "Do you want an ice cream or a milkshake?" However, if she is at the two-word level and can say "Want ice cream" then asking, "Do you want ice cream or a milkshake?" could be too limiting. A more appropriate question might be "What do you want for dessert?"

Asking questions of partners at Level 2

Partners who communicate at Level 2 are limited in their ability both to understand and to express themselves. When interacting with partners at this level, questions are frequently used to:

- confirm or interpret their messages
- let them know that they are expected to respond
- focus their attention and encourage a response

The easiest questions for partners at this level to respond to during conversations are those that require **an action response**. These are especially effective when asked during familiar events, such as getting ready to go to work.

For example, you may ask the following types of questions, using gestures to make your meaning clear:

Can I have the phone now? (hand extended toward the phone)
See the squirrel? (point to squirrel)
Will you come shopping with me? (keys in hand, point to car)
Should we go outside now? (hold door open)
Which finger should we put nail polish on first? (hold nail polish brush out)
Where does this go? (hold up framed picture)

Donald, who is at Level 2, communicates non-intentionally through facial expressions, body movement, reaching and vocalizing.

Norma, Donald's facilitator, uses a questioning intonation *to confirm and interpret his messages* when they have a conversation before breakfast:

DONALD: Begins to vocalize and heads for the kitchen.
NORMA: Follows Donald into the kitchen. ***"Hungry? Are you hungry?"***
DONALD: Sits at the table.
NORMA: Holds cereal box up to her face. ***"Cereal? D'you want cereal?"***
DONALD: Reaches for the box — action response.
NORMA: *"Yes, you are hungry."*

Now Norma asks Donald a question *to let him know that he is expected to respond.*

Norma and Donald are walking to the car, which is locked.

DONALD: Pulls at car door handle. Norma watches.
NORMA: Shows Donald the key. **"Open? Should I open the door?"**
DONALD: Continues to try to open the door.
NORMA: Moves into Donald's line of vision and waits while Donald continues trying.
DONALD: Takes Norma's hand and moves it to the door.
NORMA: *"Open. Let's open the door."* Unlocks door with the key.

In the next example, Norma asks a question with enthusiasm and expectation *to focus Donald's attention and encourage a response.*

Donald's parents are due to visit. Donald and Norma are in the living room, watching TV when the doorbell rings. Donald does not react.

NORMA: **"Was that the doorbell?"** Leans forward expectantly.
DONALD: Looks at her and smiles.
NORMA: **"Is it Mom . . . and Dad?"**
DONALD: Heads for the door and vocalizes.
NORMA: *"Let's go and see."*

Asking questions of partners at Level 3

Judy, who is at Level 3, communicates intentionally and understands quite a few words and simple instructions. She answers questions and communicates by using eye gaze, pointing, by making sounds and by gesturing. She is able to print a limited number of words, as well as to say a few words, which are not pronounced clearly.

Judy is able to understand many of the questions she is asked. However, her ability to respond with words is limited; therefore, it is best to ask questions to which she can provide some response, either through actions or through the words she can say. If they are not overused or misused, questions that require a "yes" or "no" answer can be useful because these enable Judy to stay in the conversation and to contribute constructively. For example, she can tell you whether she wants something or not, whether something happened or not and whether she agrees with something or not.

Maureen, Judy's facilitator, asks her questions *that offer her choices and opportunities to make decisions.*

Maureen has a plate with toast in one hand and a package of crackers in the other. She offers these to Judy.

MAUREEN:	***"Judy, would you like toast or crackers?"***
JUDY:	Points to the crackers, makes a sound.
MAUREEN:	Hands her the crackers. *"You always take the crackers!"*

Judy and Maureen are preparing a salad.

MAUREEN:	*"We have to do two things — first wash the lettuce and then dry it in the spinner.* **What do you want to do?"**
JUDY:	Turns on the faucet and takes a leaf of lettuce. *"Ush."*
MAUREEN:	*"Okay, you wash the lettuce and I'll dry it."*

Maureen and Judy are in Judy's bedroom. Judy's bed has been stripped and needs clean sheets.

MAUREEN:	***"Judy, what do we need?"***
JUDY:	Goes to the linen closet to get sheets.
MAUREEN:	*"Right, sheets!"*
JUDY:	*"Eee."*
MAUREEN:	*"These sheets smell so fresh."* Smells sheets.

Maureen and Judy are relaxing together and she takes the opportunity *to ask Judy questions about ongoing events.*

Judy is involved in one of her favourite activities, which is scribbling letters on a piece of paper. Maureen sits beside her and points to one of Judy's letter combinations on the page.

MAUREEN:	***"What's that?"***
JUDY:	Lifts up her purse to show Maureen.
MAUREEN:	*"Oh, that says 'purse'.* **Is that a new purse?"**
JUDY:	*"Yuh."*
MAUREEN:	***"Is there anything inside it?"***
JUDY:	*"Yuh."* Opens purse to show Maureen some money and a brush.
MAUREEN:	*"Oh, you've got some money and a brush.* **Is there anything else in there?"**
JUDY:	Shakes her head and puts the purse away.

Maureen wants to get involved with scribbling too.

MAUREEN:	Looks around. ***"Where's the other pencil?"***
JUDY:	Points to the table.
MAUREEN:	*"Okay, I see it on the table."*

The point of Judy's pencil breaks off.

MAUREEN:	Points to the broken pencil. ***"What happened? Did it break?"***
JUDY:	*"Yuh."*
MAUREEN:	***"Can you sharpen it?*** *The sharpener is over there."*
JUDY:	Goes to sharpen her pencil.

Someone is watching Judy and Maureen as they are printing.

JUDY:	Turns to look at the person watching them.
MAUREEN:	Looks at Judy. ***"Who's that?"***
JUDY:	Points.
MAUREEN:	*"That's Sam.* ***Do you know Sam?"***
JUDY:	*"Yuh."*

It is important to give your partner a chance to express herself as fully as she is able. Therefore, when you ask her a question, wait for her to answer. Give her a chance to either show you what she means or to use the few words in her vocabulary. It is also important to vary the questions you ask her and to avoid using the same ones again and again.

Asking questions of partners at Level 4

Tom communicates at Level 4 and is beginning to ask questions, such as "Whasat?" and "Where's Tina?"

Tom is verbal and so you can expect answers to your questions. However, although his vocabulary is increasing, at times he's hard to understand. Because he is talking about things which have happened in the recent past or which are not visible, you can begin to ask questions about events and people who are not present. You can even ask questions that challenge him to extend his thinking and that tap into his increased vocabulary.

Ask questions that *allow Tom to make choices.*

For example:
"Which cassette should we play?"
"Which magazine do you want to read?"
"Which way do you want to go?"

Ask Tom *about events in his life.*

For example:
> *"Where did you go today?"*
> *"What did you do there?"*
> *"Who did you see?"*

Ask Tom *to explain things to you.*

For example:
> *"What are you doing?"*
> *"What's that for?"*
> *"Why are you throwing that away?"*

Ask Tom *to clarify something you don't understand.*

For example:
> TOM: *"Tedda."*
> DAVE: (facilitator): ***"Tedda?"***
> TOM: *"Tedda."* Pulls at Dave's sweater.
> DAVE: *"Oh, sweater! You want your sweater."*

Asking questions of partners at Levels 5 and 6

Adrienne communicates at Level 5. She is able to speak in phrases and short, incomplete sentences and can provide information about familiar things and activities. Adrienne's twin, Florie, speaks mostly in short, simple sentences. Florie communicates at Level 6.

Adrienne and Florie can be asked the same types of question.

Ask Adrienne *about past events.*

For example:
> *"What did you do last night?"*
> *"How was the movie?"*
> *"What was the movie about?"*
> *"Who did you see there?"*

Ask Adrienne *to explain something to you.*

For example:
> *"Why aren't you going with Florie to see your aunt?"*
> *"How did you get your VCR to work?"*

Ask Florie *about something in the future or about future possibilities.*

For example:
> *"Where are you going for your next trip?"*
> *"What will you do on your birthday?"*

Ask Florie *to imagine.*

For example:
> *"What would you do if you won a million dollars?"*

Although Donald, Judy, Tom, Adrienne and Florie differ in their ability to communicate, appropriate questions are an effective way to keep the conversation going with all of them.

KEEP the conversation going: Use signals to encourage your partner to take another turn

Sometimes, even when you wait, show your interest and ask appropriate questions, your partner may not respond. Alternatively, she may begin the conversation well, but after taking a few turns, she may not continue. There are a few possible explanations for this: she may not realize that she is supposed to take a turn or she may not know what the appropriate turn is. Therefore, you have to make it more obvious to her — by using an appropriate signal.

Signals can be both verbal and nonverbal, and most people use a combination of these to let their partner know that she is expected to take a turn.

Verbal signals may involve:

Prompting — using cues like "Look", "Okay", "Your turn", or "Tell me what's happening?"

Repeating what you have said — using a questioning intonation or saying it louder and more slowly.

Saying the same thing in a different way — e.g., "We're going to go shopping. We're going to buy you some new clothes."

Making your question more specific — e.g., change "Are you hungry?" to "Do you want an apple?"

Changing a comment into a question — e.g., change "It's time to go to work." to "Go to work now?"

Shortening the message — e.g., change "Get washed up because we're going to visit your Mom in a few minutes." to "Wash up, then we'll go see Mom!"

You will probably find that using verbal and nonverbal signals together will help your partner understand what you have said and will enable her to respond better. It's important to wait and to give her a chance to respond to your signals. If she doesn't respond, repeat the signal or change it. Assume that you have not been clear enough and that she needs more help from you before she feels able to take her turn.

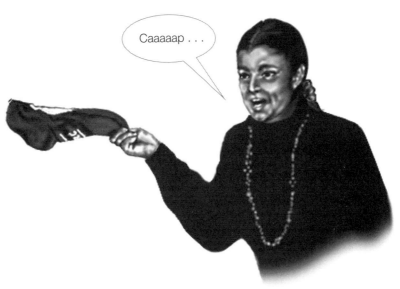

This facilitator asks her partner what he is looking for and gets no response. She thinks he may be looking for his cap, which she saw lying on the floor. So she gets the cap, asks again what he is looking for and *signals by silently mouthing the word,* while holding out the cap.

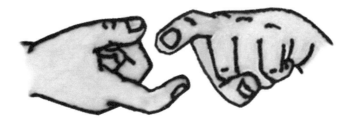

A non-verbal signal may involve *positioning your hands as if you are about to use the sign.*

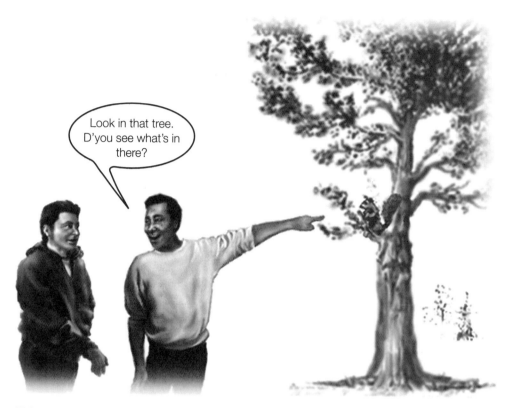

This partner didn't respond when his facilitator said, "Look what's in the tree." So he added a non-verbal signal and *pointed* at the squirrel.

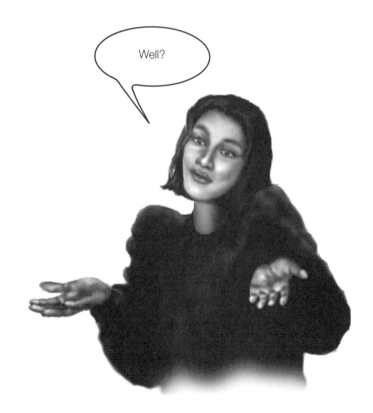

This non-verbal signal of *shrugging your shoulders and gesturing in a way that says, "Well, I'm waiting for you to respond"*, sends a clear message to your partner that she is expected to take a turn.

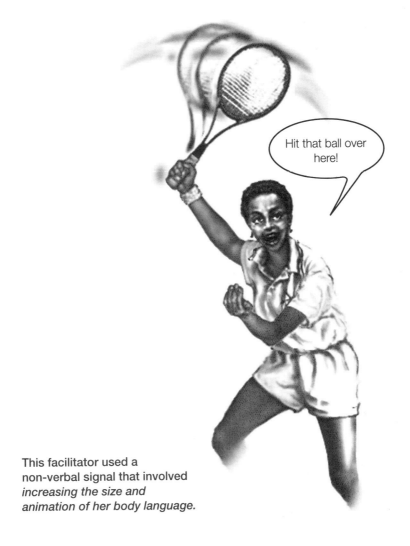

Hit that ball over here!

This facilitator used a non-verbal signal that involved *increasing the size and animation of her body language.*

REMEMBER . . . It's important to wait and to give your partner a chance to respond to your signals. If she doesn't respond, assume that you have not been clear enough and that she needs more help from you before she feels able to take her turn. Repeat the signals or change them.

LET'S REVIEW

Conversations do not have to be entirely verbal. A person's turn can be:

- a look
- facial expression
- a gesture
- a sound
- a point

You can *get* the conversation going by:

- initiating it yourself
- being face-to-face with your partner
- waiting, observing and listening to your partner so she can initiate the conversation

You can *keep* the conversation going by:

- showing your pleasure and interest
- using questions that are appropriate, genuine and at your partner's level
- using non-verbal and verbal signals to help your partner take a turn

Chapter Five # Add Information and Experience: Help Your Partner Become a Better Communicator

In the previous chapters, you learned how to share activities and keep the conversation going with your partner. Your partner's next step to becoming a better conversation partner involves learning to communicate more effectively. He needs to learn to send clearer messages, to use more sophisticated vocabulary and grammar and to talk about new topics, including those that go beyond everyday experience. What he is able to learn will depend on what he already knows and understands. However, he will learn only by interacting with someone like you, who models language appropriately during everyday conversation. Your language models will not only help him learn to express himself better, they will also enrich his understanding of language. Enriched comprehension skills lead to a better understanding of the world which, quite naturally, will give your partner more to talk about. This too, is part of becoming a more effective communicator.

In this chapter you will learn:

- how to add information and experience that promotes your partner's understanding of language as well as his ability to express himself

- to add language and experience appropriate to your partner's level of communication development

- to add information and experience at a time when your partner can best absorb it

HOW TO ADD INFORMATION AND EXPERIENCE

- Use gestures
- Use labels
- Emphasize key words
- Talk about what is happening
- Repeat — and use consistent labels
- Expand on your partner's message: Add one more word, idea or action
- Extend the topic: Build your partner's understanding of the world

Use gestures

Gestures come naturally to us; we shiver, we shake our heads, we shrug. They are an effective and often overlooked way of helping people understand language.

Gestures:

Give information — for example, you pretend to turn a steering wheel to let your partner know you are going out in your car

Show emotion — for example, you raise your hands to your cheeks to register surprise

Convey rejection or acceptance — for example, you turn your back or push something away to indicate refusal and you put your hand out to indicate acceptance

Gestures also provide the person who does not talk with a way of **expressing** himself. When you act out a message, for example, by waving to say "Goodbye" or by yawning and stretching to say "I'm tired," you are showing your partner how he could communicate.

When using gestures in everyday conversations with your partner, it is important to combine them with spoken language. This helps him learn the words which the gestures represent. At some time in the future, the gesture may serve as a "bridge" to his learning to use these words himself.

Your partner will benefit most from your use of gestures when you:

- are face-to-face with him
- say the word and make the gesture **simultaneously**
- are consistent in the words you pair with the gesture
- repeat both the words and the gesture to help him remember them

*R*emember *Holly on page 56, who communicates at Level 3 using gestures? Jean, her facilitator, knows that Holly gets very involved in interactions when Jean models gestures at the same time as she provides her with appropriate language models.*

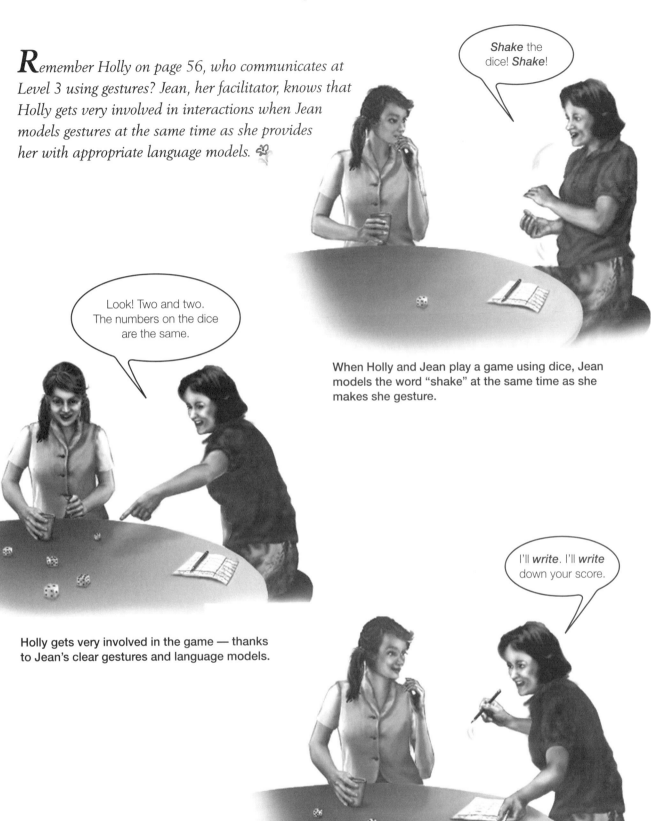

Shake the dice! *Shake*!

When Holly and Jean play a game using dice, Jean models the word "shake" at the same time as she makes she gesture.

Look! Two and two. The numbers on the dice are the same.

Holly gets very involved in the game — thanks to Jean's clear gestures and language models.

I'll *write*. I'll *write* down your score.

Jean models the gesture for "write" at the same time as she says the word. From exposure to Jean's models, Holly will learn how *she* can use gestures to participate in the game.

Use labels

In normal adult conversation, we don't need to repeat labels more than once or twice because we know that the listener knows what we are talking about. We can't, however, make the same assumption about people with limited language skills. In their case, we should assume that they need to hear specific labels again and again, either because they don't yet understand what the labels mean or because they are not yet able to express the ideas themselves.

With this in mind, think about which of the following two exchanges would better help your partner learn the word "potatoes".

This one . . .

. . . or this one?

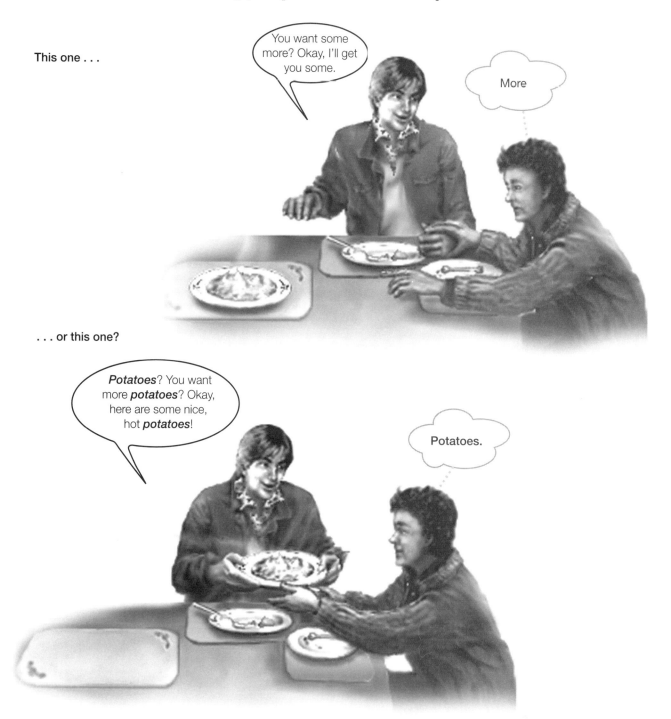

The second example obviously gives your partner much more information and helps him understand as well as learn to use the word "potato". To help him expand his vocabulary, you need to minimize your use of non-specific words like "it", "this", "that" and "some". While this will probably require a conscious effort on your part, it is well worth the trouble because your use of specific labels dramatically increases your partner's opportunities to learn new words.

Emphasize key words

When you emphasize key words in short, simple sentences, you help your partner in two ways. First, you help him identify the most important words in the sentence, and second, you help him understand the words and learn to use them. If your partner is at the earliest stages of language development, it is helpful to use two- to three-word sentences when talking to him, particularly when you are teaching him new words.

For example, Brian, John's facilitator, emphasizes the key word "Jello" five times in a variety of short, simple phrases, which are geared to John's communication at early Level 3.

BRIAN (facilitator):	*"Look, John. **Jello**."*
JOHN:	Looks.
BRIAN:	*"Your favourite. **Jello**."*
JOHN:	Looks, smiles.
BRIAN:	*"Want some **Jello**?"*
JOHN:	Leans forward slightly.
BRIAN:	*"Strawberry **Jello**."* Gives John a spoonful in his dish.
JOHN:	Eats Jello, looks at Brian.
BRIAN:	*"Mmmm, good **Jello**."*

Once John learns the meaning of "Jello", Brian will be able to use the word in longer, more natural sentences that are still within John's understanding. For example, he might say "I like Jello too," or "Wow! This Jello is slippery!"

Brian can also highlight and exaggerate key words by:

Pausing before the key word — "Want . . . Jello?"

Prolonging the key word — "Jeeeeello".

Varying loudness — whispering "Jello" or saying "JELLO" loudly.

Drawing attention to what is being talked about — by pointing to or holding up the bowl of "Jello".

If your partner speaks at the single word or two-word stage, you should speak in short, simple sentences, emphasizing the words he is likely to be able to imitate. And when accompanying your language with signs which you want your partner to imitate, sign only the words that are key to your message.

Talk about what is happening

It is important to talk about what you and your partner are doing as it happens. This is like taking a "verbal walk" through an activity. Even if your partner knows what action comes next — such as putting a dish into a cupboard once it's dry — he may not have the language to correspond with the action. When you talk about something of interest to your partner as it is happening, language becomes much more concrete and interesting for him.

It is important to be aware that your partner's receptive language (what he understands) is likely to be more advanced than his expressive language (what he can say or sign). This will affect the complexity of your language.

If you expect your partner to imitate what you say — speak at his expressive language level.

If you are talking about ongoing activities and events, with no expectation that your partner will imitate you — gear your language to his receptive language level. If he is able to understand a great deal more than he can express, talk to him using more complex sentences.

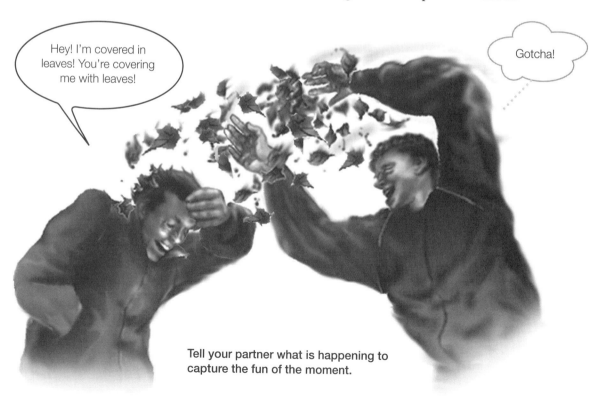

Hey! I'm covered in leaves! You're covering me with leaves!

Gotcha!

Tell your partner what is happening to capture the fun of the moment.

Repeat — and use consistent labels

At first, your partner may not be able to understand, say or sign the words you use in your daily routines and activities. However, as he hears the words paired again and again with the people, things and events they represent, he will come to understand them. When the words and gestures become predictable to your partner, he stands a better chance of learning to use them.

How many times do you need to repeat a word or sign before your partner will try to imitate it? Some people need 10 repetitions of a word, gesture or sign before they will attempt it; others need hundreds. Your task is to find several ways to use the same word in many different situations.

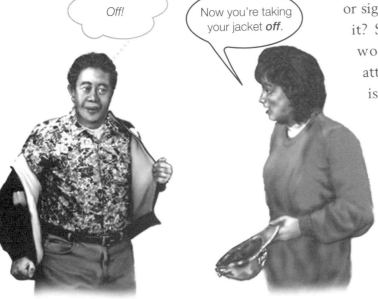

An alert facilitator makes a point of modelling the same word . . . .

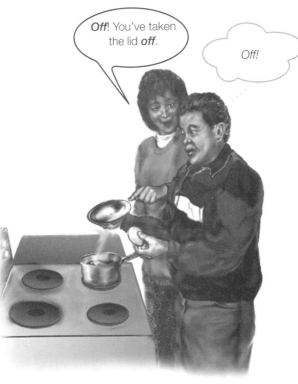

. . . again and again . . .

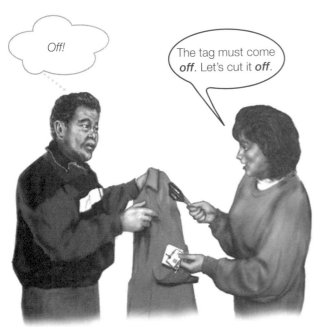

. . . in many different situations.

Expand on your partner's message: Add one more word, idea or action

It is important to keep your language simple when conversing with people who have limited language skills, but it's also critical to show them the next step. This can be done by **expanding** on your partner's message.

Expanding involves adding a small amount of information to your partner's message. This gives him the chance to hear and see new words, signs or symbols in relation to the topic of the conversation. When expanding is coupled with gestures and an emphasis on key words, it promotes your partner's expressive and receptive language skills at the same time.

One of the easiest ways to help your partner develop more mature language is to:

Say what your partner says — and add **one more word**; or,

Say what your partner says — and **add one more idea** to the topic;

and/or

Do what your partner does — and **add one more gesture or action**

The expanded information should:

- be slightly above your partner's expressive level – i.e. it should provide him with a model of a slightly more advanced way of expressing himself
- be clearly related to what he has said
- be interesting and relatively easy to understand
- be highlighted so that it stands out from the rest of the words
- contain gestures, words or ideas that he would be motivated to use himself

Expanding is the key to building your partner's expressive and receptive communication skills. It is important to think carefully about how you expand so you are neither too far below nor too far above his level. This means keeping the added information relatively simple for partners at Levels 3 and 4, while using more complex information for partners at higher levels of communication.

Expanding for your partner at Level 2

Your partner, Nancy: Heads for the door
You **imitate** and add **one**:
- **to the action**: You walk to the door, place your hand on the doorknob and wait expectantly; and then you add:
- **to the topic**: *"**Out!** You want **out!**"*

Expanding for your partner at Level 3

Marie: Points to a flower and says, "Fwaw!"

You **imitate** (by modelling the correct form of the word) **and**:

- **add one more word**: *"Flower. Pretty flower."*

To make the conversation more interesting, you can smell the flower and:

- **add one more idea**: *"Flower. It smells nice";* and combine this with
- **one more gesture or action**: Sniff or pretend to sniff the flower.

Expanding for your partner at Level 4

Howard: Points to the picture symbol for "Wash hands."

You **imitate** (point to the picture) and **add one**:

- to the sentence: *"You want to wash hands."*

Then you can expand his understanding of language by adding:

- to the **topic**: *"Your hands are dirty."* (pointing to the dirt).

Expanding for your partner at Level 5

Leah: *"Betty a baby."*

You imitate and add:

- to the sentence: *"Did Betty have a baby?"*

And then, to improve Leah's understanding of language, add:

- to the topic: *"So Michael has a new sister."*

Expanding for your partner at Level 6

John: *"I'm working on this."*

You add:

- to the sentence: *"You're working really hard on it."*

And then, to improve John's understanding of language, add:

- to the topic: *"You're taking the whole motor apart."*

REMEMBER . . . The most language learning will occur when your response is related to your partner's focus of interest or to what he has communicated.

*J*oan *has Down Syndrome and is a Level 4 communicator who is attracted to colour and movement. Her facilitator, Barbara, thinks it is a perfect day for blowing bubbles outside. Joan readily follows Barbara outside when she gestures and says, "Come on". Barbara starts blowing bubbles through the wand, and* *when Joan sees the bubbles rise into the air, her excitement is unmistakable. Now Barbara has the perfect opportunity to expand on what Joan communicates, making this a powerful language learning activity.*

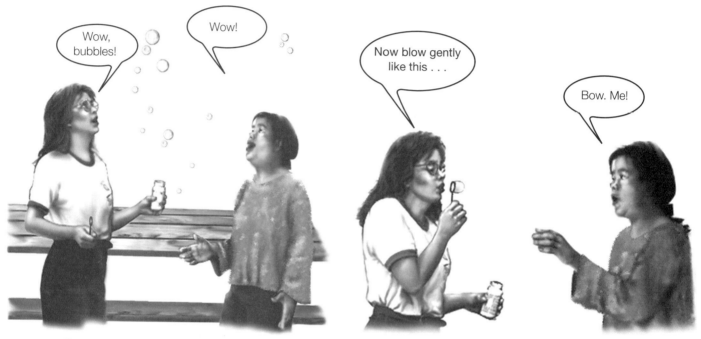

Barbara imitates Joan and adds one more word.

Barbara describes how she blows the bubbles, and Joan wants to try.

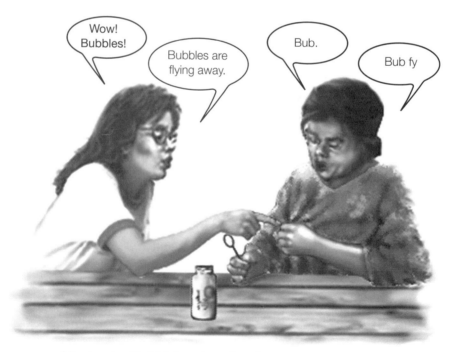

After hearing "bubble" again and again, Joan imitates it. Then Barbara expands, capturing Joan's focus, and Joan responds again.

Stay tuned — there's more to this story later on in the chapter!

Extend the topic: Build your partner's understanding of the world

Many of your partners at Levels 4, 5 and 6 have receptive abilities that far exceed their abilities to express themselves. It is important for them to be exposed to information that will enrich their understanding of language and of the world, even if they are not able to express all of these themselves. The only way they can expand on their ability to express themselves is through ongoing exposure to more abstract language during conversations.

You can extend the topic when either you or your partner initiates, but you will need to judge what to say depending on his level of understanding.

You can **describe** — e.g., if your partner sees someone with a newborn baby, you can say, "That baby is so tiny. Look at his tiny fingers."

You can **explain** — e.g., if your partner can't get a flashlight to work, you can say, "I think the batteries are dead. The flashlight won't work because the batteries are so old."

You can **talk about feelings** — e.g., if your partner looks upset because his parents haven't arrived to pick him up, you can say, "You're sad. Your parents aren't here yet."

You can **project into situations never experienced or into others' reactions to experiences** — e.g., when the two of you are looking at a newspaper article about a space shuttle, you can say, "Those astronauts must feel so excited to be in space."

You can **talk about the future** — e.g., if your partner is listening to someone talking about a vacation, you can say, "Soon you'll be going on vacation. You're going camping in the summer. "

You can **imagine** — e.g., when your partner starts to sing while you are taking a walk, you can pretend to give him a microphone, pretend to hold one yourself and say, "Ladies and gentleman, introducing John Gardiner, the famous singer from Mapleville, Canada!" and clap your hands.

Many people with developmental delays have difficulty understanding language, especially abstract language. Your sensitive efforts to extend the topic by describing, explaining, talking about feelings, projecting, talking about the future and imagining will expand your partner's knowledge and understanding and show him how this kind of language can be used in everyday conversations.

*J*oan and Barbara from page 87 are still outdoors, having fun blowing bubbles. Joan continues to be fascinated with them. As she watches them float into the air, she repeats "Bub" from time to time. Barbara begins describing the bubbles and uses repetition to help Joan understand what she is saying. She says things like: "Look at the bubbles!", "So many bubbles.", "There's a big bubble!", "That bubble popped." then she extends the topic . . .

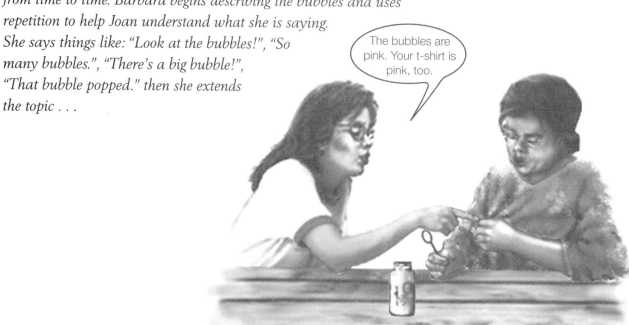

Barbara extends the topic by describing the bubbles.

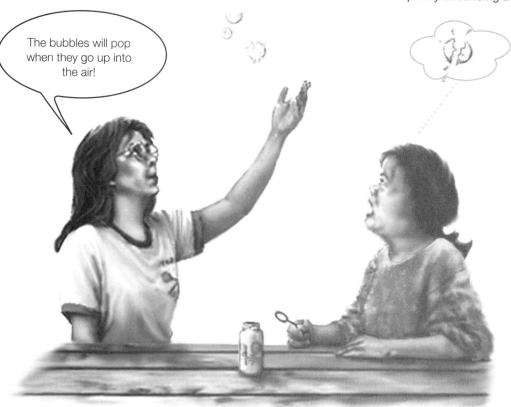

She extends the topic by talking about the future.

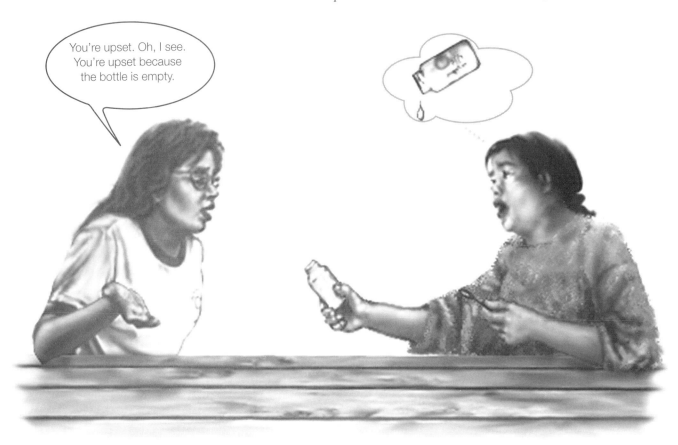

Barbara extends the topic by talking about Joan's feelings and explaining that the jar is empty.

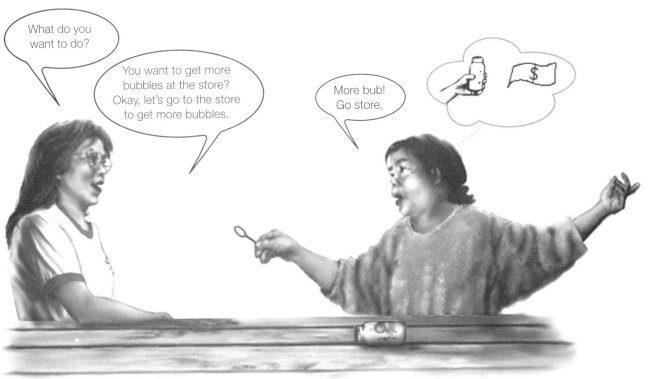

Barbara provides Joan with a correct model and then agrees to go to the store, allowing Joan to experience the power of communication.

ADD LANGUAGE AND EXPERIENCE APPROPRIATE TO YOUR PARTNER'S LEVEL OF COMMUNICATION

How to add language when your partner is at Level 1 or 2

When your partner communicates at Level 1, you interpret his sounds, facial expressions and body language. His smiles, cries, screams and movements succeed in communicating his feelings and needs to you.

At Levels 1 and 2, although your partner is still not communicating in a conventional way, you can interpret his facial expressions, body language and sounds as he begins to reach out and connect with the environment.

When your partner is at Level 1 or 2, you play a critical role in helping him become **aware** of other people and of the power and pleasure of communication. This is what leads him to become **intentional**.

When adding language and experience for your partner at Level 1 or 2, you can:

- imitate your partner's sounds and actions; then add something new
- use gestures
- interpret — say it as he would if he could
- show him the objects you are talking about
- wait for a response — any response
- name people and label things in which he shows an interest
- talk in simple sentences about what's happening
- emphasize key words
- repeat — and use labels consistently

How to add language when your partner is at Level 3

At Level 3, your partner is interested in connecting with those around him. He looks at you to make sure you are paying attention to what interests him. He intentionally sends messages, using many different ways to communicate. He uses a few words or signs, but mostly he points, uses body language, gestures and actions, and makes sounds that stand for words. Messages are simple and are sent one idea at a time. He is also able to understand some of what he hears.

When adding language and experience for your partner at Level 3, you can:

- interpret — "paste" simple spoken language over his nonverbal message, capturing his focus and intent
- emphasize key words that your partner may be able to imitate and express

- imitate his non-verbal communication and then expand — add simple information which he can understand
- talk about what is happening, about the people, events, objects and actions in the environment
- repeat — and be consistent

How to add language when your partner is at Level 4, 5 or 6

At Levels 4, 5 and 6 your partner uses words, signs/symbols and phrases consistently, even if they are hard to understand. You can continue to help him understand and say more so that his messages become more conventional, easier to understand and increasingly more complex.

When adding language and experience for your partner at Levels 4, 5 and 6 you can:

- emphasize key words
- keep expanding — add longer comments on the topic
- link your partner's comment to his past experience
- talk about what is happening
- extend the topic, exposing him to more abstract language

TAKE ADVANTAGE OF THE BEST TIMES TO ADD INFORMATION

Add information:
- when your partner wants something
- during daily routines
- when things go wrong
- when your partner's initiations are undesirable

Add information when your partner wants something

When your partner wants something, capture the moment! These are the times when he will be most receptive to the information you provide.

These moments allow you to:

- take advantage of his captured attention
- respond immediately to encourage him to take another turn
- model the appropriate gestures, words, signs and/or picture symbols while maintaining eye contact with him
- give him what he wants, but only after holding onto it for a few seconds.
- add information at his level

*S*andy, an experienced facilitator, works with Nate, who communicates non-verbally at early Level 3. He is a man with his own agenda, who enjoys sensory experiences. However, Sandy has learned to make the most of those moments when Nate wants something. 🌿

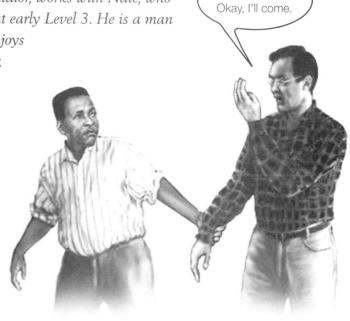

When Nate pulls on Sandy's hand, Sandy interprets and shows him how to use the appropriate gesture.

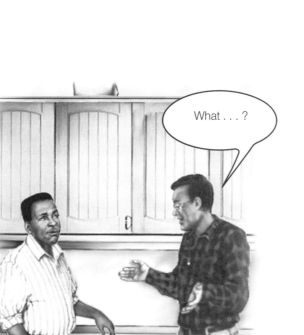

Nate takes Sandy to the cupboards, then stands and looks at him. Sandy, who knows what Nate wants, waits expectantly for a clearer message.

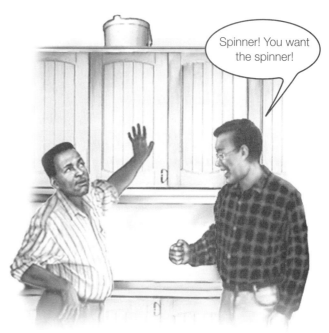

Nate then bangs on the cupboard door where the salad spinner is kept. He uses this for his favourite activity — making the salad spinner spin and then removing its lid so he can watch the basket whirl around. Sandy immediately responds, taking the opportunity to interpret Nate's message and to add a gesture that conveys "spinning".

Add information during daily routines

Daily routines are a prime time for language learning because the same words are repeated every day in familiar situations.

You and your partner probably spend a lot of time sharing the following routines of daily life:

- washing
- grooming
- mealtime
- putting on jackets, coats, etc.
- dressing
- brushing teeth
- applying make-up
- coffee breaks

You may also share some of the following activities:

- unloading the dryer
- opening mail
- washing the car
- setting the table
- baking
- renting movies
- buying groceries
- shovelling snow
- washing dishes
- making beds
- writing letters
- banking
- putting groceries away
- raking leaves
- loading dishwasher
- preparing a meal
- exercising

Your partner will learn from these routines only if you talk about what's happening as you and he carry them out. Describe what you and he are doing as you are doing it, giving him a chance to both initiate and respond. Even if he doesn't initiate, he may become interested in joining in the conversation once you get it started — and he will learn a great deal in the process.

Add information when things go wrong

Consider things going wrong as a golden opportunity to describe and explain what has happened. Don't always try to set things right as soon as something goes wrong; use these times to build your partner's understanding of language.

*Cathy communicates at Level 4. She speaks using single words, but is hard to understand. At her day program, she frequently washes the dishes, which are unbreakable. The glasses, however, aren't. One day, Cathy shatters a glass on the floor. Margie, her facilitator, describes what has happened: "Oh, the glass **fell**. It's **broken** now." She suggests a solution: "We'd better **sweep it up**." Walking towards the broom cupboard, she says, "Let's get the **dustpan** and **broom** so we can **sweep** it up." She gives Cathy the dustpan and she begins to sweep the pieces of glass into it. Cathy tries to help by picking up a piece from the floor. Margie says, "Be careful, the pieces are **sharp**," and she points to the sharp edge. "That can **cut** you. Just throw it into the **dustpan**." Instead of simply doing the job herself, Margie turns this situation into a language learning opportunity for Cathy.*

Your partner will learn from an experience that goes wrong if you explain:

- what happened
- why it happened
- how to correct the problem

*P*atrick *(Level 4) trips and falls as he walks into a room. His facilitator's simply worded comment, "Oh, you fell," followed by an explanation, "I think the carpet is loose," and a solution, "Let's get some tools to fix it", help Patrick focus on the event (and not on his grazed knee) and on the language that goes along with it. His facilitator also invites Patrick's participation and, together, they get the tools and secure the loose carpet.*

Add information when initiations are undesirable

Sometimes your partner may say or do something which is undesirable or unsafe. "Don'ts" and refusals can be an essential part of working with some of your partners, but constant "No's" don't promote learning. When you can't allow your partner to lead, you **can** explain why not.

If initiations are unsafe	you can explain why and remove the danger
If your partner is behaving inappropriately	you can explain what he is doing wrong and show and/or tell him what would be more acceptable
If your partner has requested an activity when time is limited	you can explain that you can't do it right now, but if he wants, you can do it "later". You must then follow through so he will trust that "later" means an eventual "yes"

LET'S REVIEW

Adding information involves fine-tuning your language so your partner can move on to the next level of communication. The following non-verbal and verbal techniques will provide him with the information he needs to communicate more effectively:

Use gestures as you talk — show your partner how he can communicate in many ways through body language.

Use labels — and minimize the use of words such as "this", "that" and "it".

Emphasize key words — to help your partner focus on what is important in the message you're sending.

Talk about what is happening — take "verbal walks" around the things that command your partner's interest and/or during activities in which you and/or your partner are involved.

Repeat and use consistent labels — to maximize learning, associate the word as often as possible with the item, person or action to which it refers.

Expand: Add one more word, idea or action — add information to your partner's message by imitating his message, and then adding one more piece of information.

Extend the topic: Build your partner's understanding of the world by:

- describing
- talking about feelings
- talking about the future
- explaining
- projecting
- imagining

Add language and experience at your partner's level of communication — gear your language to your partner's level of receptive language when you are talking about what is happening and about things that are not present. But when you expect him to try to imitate you, use only words or signs that he can imitate!

Make the most of the best times to add information, such as:

- when your partner wants something
- during daily routines
- when things go wrong
- when initiations are undesirable

Chapter Six

Chapter Six

Encourage the Use of an Augmentative or Alternative Communication (AAC) System During Interactions

The 3As provide the foundation for all interactions with your partners. These A's, Allow, Adapt and Add, represent generic strategies that can be adapted for all of your partners, whether they are verbal or not. However, a special picture emerges when you interact with people who are ready to represent their ideas but whose speech is either inadequate or non-existent.

They must use augmentative or alternative communication (AAC) systems to convey their messages, and the 3A approach must accommodate this additional component.

What's the difference between augmentative and alternative systems? Although they are closely related, the terms represent a fundamental difference in the way you expect a partner to communicate. People who are able to communicate in a limited manner, and whose communication can be expanded upon by adding a more efficient system, need an **augmentative system**. For example, let's consider a person who is able to convey the following messages effectively: she can say "yes", "no", "home" and "milk"; she can sign "hungry", "more" and "mine"; she points to things she wants and points out things she likes, such as someone's clothing; she vocalizes for attention. She cannot, however, communicate other messages such as "broken" (as in "My watch is broken."), "Rent a movie" and "Stop that". Therefore, these last three ideas must be included in an augmentative system that *supplements*, but does not replace, the ideas she can already communicate using speech, sign and gesture. People who do not have access to *any* means of communication need more than an augmentative system — their system is considered **"alternative"** — and is the primary or only way they can communicate with others.

The implementation of an AAC system should be a joint effort which includes your partner, her speech-language pathologist, other support team members and yourself. Your contributions to vocabulary selection will be based on the perspective you have gained from spending time with her and will form the basis for only part of an AAC system.

Much has been written about techniques for teaching and facilitating AAC use, and those techniques will not be addressed here. This chapter will focus primarily on suggestions for the selection of appropriate vocabulary in specific shared activities for your partner so that your efforts to Allow, Adapt and Add will be effective.

In this chapter, you will learn how to add information to the AAC system that is:

F lexible

A ctive

I ndividualized

R espected

so the AAC system reflects your partner's growth throughout her lifetime and so that you encourage her to use her system consistently.

AAC SYSTEMS NEED TO BE FAIR

Although AAC systems are intended for daily use, many people who have these systems hardly use them. The reason for this is that many systems are inadequate and provide people with little motivation to use them. In addition to the inadequacies of the system itself, there are various human factors that affect the successful use of an AAC system. The addition of a third ingredient, such as a picture board, into the interactive mix between facilitator and partner can create some special reactions — and discomfort is one of them.

You may experience discomfort in using an AAC system with your partner because:

- much time and effort is spent compiling a system which your partner doesn't use
- you find yourself reverting to the "Director", "Helper" or "Mover" role in an effort to teach your partner to use the system
- you aren't familiar with the system and so you circumvent the need for your partner to use it. You may use other less interactive ways of finding out what she wants to say, such as asking questions that require only a "yes" or "no" response

Even when your partner knows and uses the system, the interaction can still break down if the words you and she need are not in her system. Your partner relies on you to provide her with the words she needs to express herself. Choosing vocabulary which she will use is a long process — one that should continue throughout her life. Ineffective vocabulary choices are among the chief culprits in communication breakdowns with AAC users. This places the onus on you to monitor the words that are available to your partner when you interact with her.

If your partner uses, or could use, augmentative or alternative communication, it is important to set her up for success. In order to be successful, AAC systems must be **FAIR**:

Flexible: the system must reflect your partner's ever-changing ability to communicate and understand and must contain vocabulary that can be used in a variety of situations

Active: the system must be capable of being used at any time

Individualized: the system must contain vocabulary that your partner wants and needs to use

Respected: the system must be perceived by your partner as valuable to the interaction between other people and herself

Add information to the AAC system that is Flexible

In an AAC system, symbols should be included that can be used in any situation. For example:

- greetings
- introductions — e.g., "My name is...."
- "yes" and "no"
- people's names
- topics your partner often talks about
- specific interests
- words with more than one meaning which your partner knows and can use often — e.g., "bark"; "clear"; "cap"
- common events — e.g., work, birthdays
- words that can be combined with other words to form new concepts — e.g., "long" and "water" to convey "river"
- phrases that allow your partner some control over the vocabulary on her display, such as "add that word to my board" or "take that word off"

Encourage **A**ctive use of your partner's system

Your partner best learns how to use an AAC system when she uses it purposefully during interactions. Her motivation to use the system will grow only if it achieves what she wants and needs it to. Therefore, when your partner uses an augmentative system, it is critical that you use the strategies described in previous chapters that keep her engaged in interactions. You need to allow her to take the lead, to adapt activities so they can be shared, to encourage conversation by adapting your behaviour and to add information fine-tuned to her level.

Yet more is needed to encourage active communication from your partner. This can be achieved if you:

- focus more on the individual than on the system
- model use of the system by using it yourself
- ask questions that allow your partner to use her vocabulary
- encourage others to speak directly to your partner

Focus more on the individual than on the system

Because an AAC system introduces another component to the interaction, you may find all your attention focused on the system rather than on your partner. To counteract this, be face-to-face as much as possible. Establish eye contact with your partner, even if you are sitting side by side.

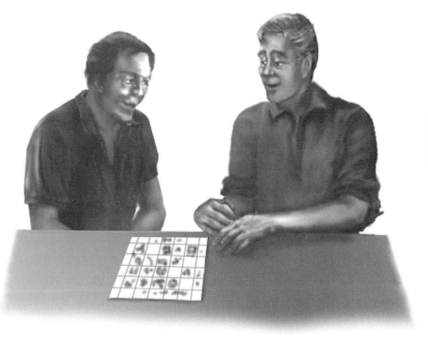

Focus more on your partner than on the display — be face-to-face as much as possible when an augmentative communication display is used.

Model use of the system by using it yourself

When you communicate with your partner, send your message in pictures or sign. There are several benefits to this practice:

- it shows your partner that using a picture system or sign language is a perfectly valid and acceptable method of communicating with others
- it is helpful in demonstrating how such a system can be used, especially when your partner is first learning to use AAC in everyday activities
- it helps you become familiar with the placement and content of the symbols on the display or with the signs
- it shows others at home or at work that the device is meant to be used during everyday interactions

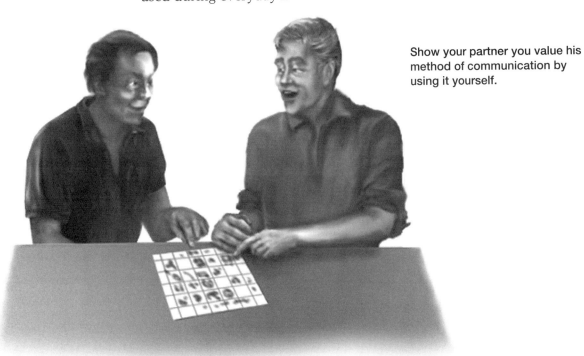

Show your partner you value his method of communication by using it yourself.

Ask questions that allow your partner to use her vocabulary

Yes-no questions are frequently overused with partners who have limited communication skills because they offer a quick way of getting information. However, if used too frequently, they send the message both to your partner and to others that her AAC system is not useful. This is a sure-fire conversation stopper that can limit your partner's ability to learn and to influence her own life.

Asking questions to which your partner can provide her own responses will help her reveal her own unique personality and preferences. For example, rather than asking, "Do you want to go for a walk to the park?", use your partner's picture board to let her tell you which of the possible activities represented on her display she would like to do.

Encourage others to speak directly to your partner

An AAC system is designed to give your partner a better way of communicating with others about a variety of topics. It can only be effective if others use it to communicate directly with her. A vital part of the success of the system involves encouraging verbal and non-verbal peers, as well as family members, staff and anyone else to speak directly to your partner — and not to use you as an intermediary.

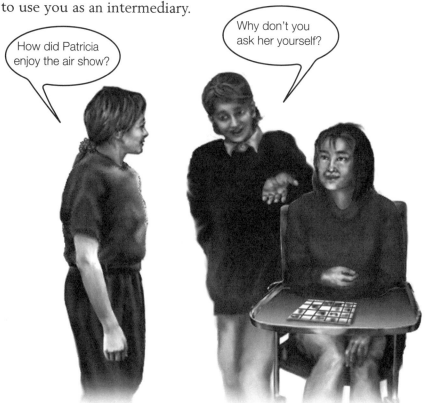

Encourage others to speak directly to the person who uses the AAC system.

Giving your partner the opportunity to speak for herself and to participate in all aspects of life helps her and others around her to see that she too has something valuable to contribute. There is nothing that will build her self-esteem more than having others view and treat her as a unique and special human being who is worthy of their attention.

Individualize vocabulary selection for your partner

Everyday interactions are fertile ground for discovering which words need to be included in your partner's system. These interactions also provide you with opportunities to provide these words for her and to see if they are useful.

Much of the guesswork in selecting appropriate vocabulary for an AAC system can be minimized by examining your partner's unique needs at each of the following stages of an interaction:

Preactive: *before* the two of you interact and communicate

Active: *while* the two of you are interacting and communicating

Reactive: *after* the two of you have completed your interaction

In some ways, selecting vocabulary for future use (preactive) is a predictive process — and you should expect that many of these predictions will fail. If you don't get it right the first time, keep trying! If your partner rejects a new vocabulary item, then the process becomes an active as well as a reactive one.

Your examination of your partner's vocabulary needs involves a dynamic cycle that continually repeats itself. This cycle maintains the focus on your partner and keeps her expressive repertoire in synchrony with all her life's experiences.

The PREACTIVE stage of vocabulary selection

Your partner may not yet have an AAC system, or she may have an outdated one. In either case, begin by listing activities which you share with your partner. When interacting with your partner, remember to:

S hare activities

L isten to what your partner is saying

O bserve your partner's behaviour

W ait — give your partner a chance to communicate

Ask yourself the following questions:

- What does my partner want to say?
- How does she convey these messages?
- What could my partner say, given a chance?
- What has my partner tried, but been unable to communicate in the past in a given situation?
- What ideas do her parents, teachers and other caregivers have about her interests and reasons for communicating in similar activities?

- What has my partner expressed about her interests in the past?
- How motivated is my partner to convey a specific message?
- Is my partner consistently communicating any message in an unsophisticated way? Could she do so in a more conventional way?

Over several weeks, keep a record of all of your partner's messages in the context of the activities you have listed. In addition, record all of the ways in which she sent these messages. This record can become your source book for ideas when you actually begin using augmentative symbols in your activities together. Talk to your partner and ask her which of the messages she wants to be included in her system. She may like your choices, or she may have something else in mind!

Sanja works in a warehouse with a group of adults who also have developmental delays. Most of them are able to speak and read better than Sanja, who is extremely difficult to understand. As a result, she speaks only when she has to, and then only in single words. However, she can understand much more than she can say. Her facilitator, Corrie, thinks that if Sanja could speak more clearly, she would have lots to say. Sanja's speech-language pathologist agrees. Because Sanja's potential to improve her speech is poor, Sanja, her family, facilitators and the speech-language pathologist agree to try a picture-based communication system, and a plan of action is devised.

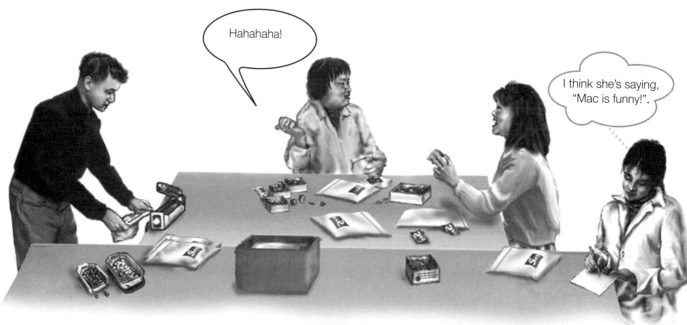

Sometimes Sanja laughs and directs her co-workers' attention to another colleague, but is unable to add anything meaningful. In the pre-active stage of collecting vocabulary, Corrie, Sanja's facilitator, records what Sanja seems to be saying.

Corrie is responsible for gathering potential vocabulary for the picture board, so she spends time observing Sanja at work. Sanja places labels on plastic bags that contain pieces of hardware. She knows where to get more labels when she runs out, and the production line is organized so that the bags are placed in front of her, ready to be labelled. There is little opportunity for Sanja to communicate while she is working.

At break time Sanja tends to sit at the table with her peers and simply listen to their conversation. She can't keep up. What she needs is a way to invite her peers to interact with her. The initial vocabulary selected for Sanja includes some of the messages which she has already tried to convey non-verbally, as well as some that could be used to engage others in conversation. Included are: "hello", "goodbye", "yes", "no", "thank you", "What have you been up to?", "You're nuts, you know", and a blank area for her parents to add information about what Sanja has done the night before.

Once the pictures have been compiled into a display, Corrie and Sanja's speech-language pathologist coach Sanja in its use. It does not take long for Sanja to catch on to the picture for "You're nuts, you know".

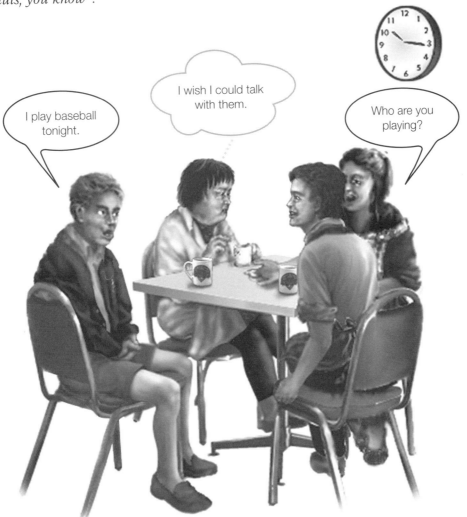

Sanja can't keep up with the conversation, so she doesn't even try to interact.

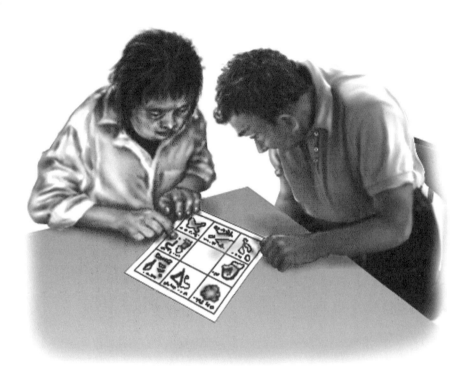

Although the vocabulary on Sanja's display may still not allow her to have a full-fledged conversation, it is an important start. But there's still a long way to go! 🪻

One of Sanja's peers is attracted to her display and begins to talk to her and ask her questions. The display allows Sanja to respond with appropriate information and to ask questions herself, a level of participation which she thoroughly enjoys.

In the preactive stage of vocabulary selection, collect the picture symbols and learn the signs that correspond with the messages you think should be included in the AAC system. Then either add them to the system before you engage in the activity or save them for future use.

The ACTIVE stage of vocabulary selection

Vocabulary selection in this stage occurs while you and your partner are involved in an activity together. The need for specific words and messages becomes especially obvious when the flow of communication breaks down and you can't understand what your partner is trying to tell you. In this case, you will have to:

- interpret or guess at your partner's message and try to get confirmation from her response.

If you figure out what her message is, ask her if this is one she would like to have in her system.

- add the information by immediately providing the picture or modelling the sign

Your partner's "need-to-know" is a prime moment to encourage learning. If the corresponding picture or sign was targeted during the preactive stage of vocabulary selection, it can be made available at this time.

- record pictures or signs for future use if you are not able to produce them immediately

Michel is a Level 4 communicator who loves going to fast food restaurants. He uses a picture book to communicate and one of the categories in his book is the local fast food restaurant. In the pre-active stage of vocabulary selection, his facilitators have tried to anticipate what he might request. Let's look at how Ned, Michel's facilitator, responds when he realizes that the picture book is missing something Michel needs.

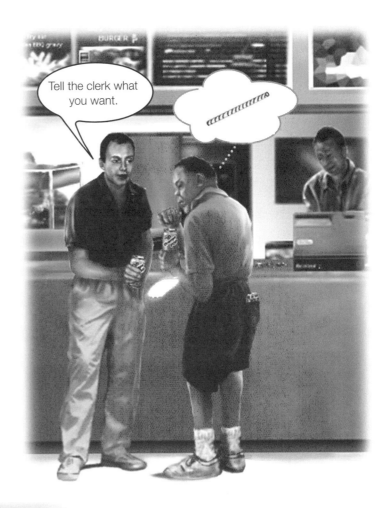

While Michel and Ned are in the local fast food restaurant, they each order a cold drink. Michel looks around, but he can't see any straws.

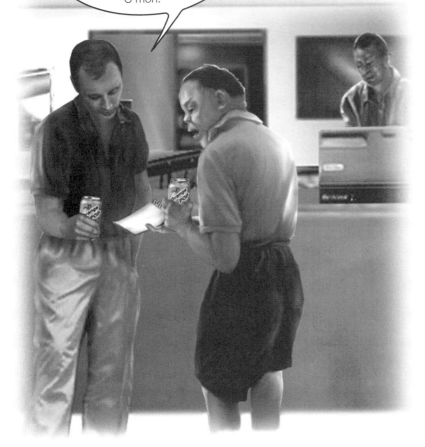

Ned knows it's important not to speak for Michel. He and Michel search the picture book for a picture symbol of a straw, but it's not there.

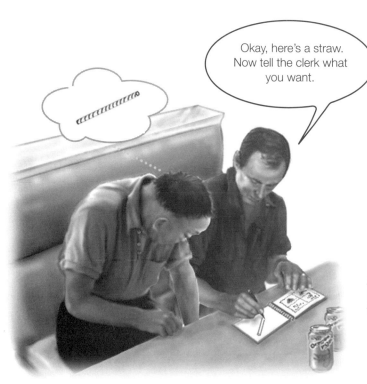

Ned's determination to keep Michel's display useful and updated is obvious. He takes advantage of concrete opportunities to encourage Michel to communicate with someone he hardly knows — leaving Michel feeling the glow of success. ❧

Although Ned keeps extra symbols on hand, he doesn't have one for "straw". But Ned is flexible and so he draws one.

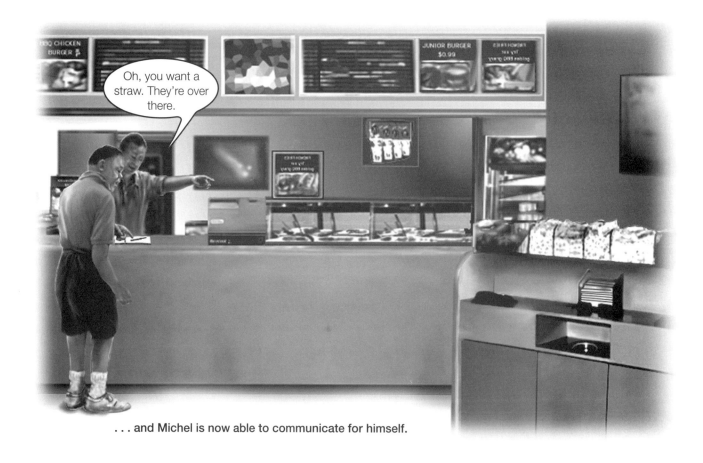

. . . and Michel is now able to communicate for himself.

The REACTIVE stage of vocabulary selection

Sometimes, all your best guesses before — and even during — the activity do not help you figure out the words your partner needs. When she tries to tell you something, either you cannot understand it or she lets you know, in some way, that the words are not in her repertoire.

Once the activity is over, you need to take time to evaluate what has happened. Sometimes, just giving yourself a chance to stop and think can help you see the messages you might have missed. Ask yourself what you were doing during the activity. Could your behaviour have triggered an unintelligible string of sounds, gestures and movements from your partner? Could she have wanted to do something different during the activity? Possibly she was trying to tell you about something other than the activity. You may have to ask other people who live and work with her to discover what she might have been trying to convey.

The answers to these questions can be a rich source of useful vocabulary for your partner. The use of such vocabulary can be facilitated on a "need-to-know" basis or can be systematically taught in a formalized program of instruction. It is only by trial and error that you will find a repertoire of words that will work for your partner.

A family of elderly brothers all communicate in the same way. They are very sociable — they gesture and speak using adult intonation, but their speech is extremely difficult to understand. They can call for attention ("Hey!"), agree and disagree ("Yeah" and "No") and are able to use other single words that pop up every now and then. Facilitators who know them well understand what they are trying to say from the consistency of their intonations, gestures and sounds as well as from knowing what is happening in their lives.

Last summer, they had a visitor (a speech-language pathologist) at the centre where they spend their days. After greeting her, Clark, one of the brothers, started gesturing to her, making a circle with his arms out in front of him. Amidst the jargon, the words "Round! Round!" could be made out. He then pointed behind him, saying "Over there!" "Something round is over there?" tried the speech-language pathologist. "No," responded Clark, and repeated the message. "Oh," said his facilitator, "he's telling you that today he and his brothers are going to the park that has the carousel."

Another brother, Harvey, approached the visitor. He pointed out the window and began to chatter. The words "Over there" could be made out, but again, the message was unclear. Again the speech-language pathologist felt helpless, and the facilitator had to come to her rescue. "He's telling you that our centre is moving," she explained. "Yeah," Harvey confirmed, and chattered again. "Right," the supervisor agreed, "next month." "Yeah," came Harvey's reply.

The visitor accompanied the brothers to the park. When they returned to the centre, she and the brothers sat down around a communication device that provides speech when activated. Between the visitor and two of the four brothers, picture symbols were selected and messages were programmed into the machine about what they had done at the park and about the centre's move. They then practised activating the messages, which the brothers really enjoyed. Following this, the brothers showed off their newfound skills with the communication device when they took it home and communicated the events of their day to their facilitators.

Respect your partner's system

You can help and encourage your partner and those who spend time with her to develop a positive attitude toward using her AAC system in the following ways:

- resist the temptation to speed up the process of communication
- make the AAC system available at all times
- keep the system up to date
- adapt the system so it's accessible

Resist the temptation to speed up the process of communication

If you find that your partner is slow in using her AAC system, if time is short and you are beginning to get anxious — don't despair! It's very normal to experience such frustration and to want to speed up the process by using quicker (but less interactive) methods such as questions which require only a "yes" or "no" response.

But resist the temptation. More is accomplished when you take the time to allow your partner to use her system. This is *her* voice, and she deserves to be heard.

Make the AAC system available at all times

Be sure your partner's AAC is available to her at all times. Wait for her to use her board when it is her turn to communicate. Allow her to lead, and check your tendency to jump in, help her or speak for her. She must communicate for herself — she's the only one who knows what she wants to say!

Keep the AAC system up to date

People's circumstances and interests change over time and, consequently, so will their vocabulary needs. One AAC display can never be adequate over the course of your partner's entire lifetime.

Those who rely on others to make their language available to them through an AAC system must also count on these people to be aware of and to adapt to any changes in their lives. Symbols in the system should be adjusted as needed and on a regular basis. Include new symbols as the circumstances of your partner's life change and drop those that are never used.

Adapt the AAC system so it's accessible

We have learned to accommodate people with different challenges. We build ramps for people in wheelchairs, we use Braille on elevator buttons for those with visual impairments and we use teletype telephones and flashing lights for people with hearing impairments.

People with different communication abilities also require accommodations that are their "ramps" to communication. People who sign need a signing community around them — facilitators, friends and family who can use and understand sign language. People who use picture symbol communication also need us to make adaptions so that their symbols are accessible and accepted.

Some topics of conversation require words that are specific to certain situations and environments. For example, when talking about eating or cooking meals, it is highly likely that vocabulary relating to the kitchen will be needed. When talking about grocery shopping, depending on the tastes of the people involved, there are likely to be many predictable "food" words. When talking about household chores such as making beds, vocabulary will once again be fairly predictable, since sheets and blankets all have to be changed regularly, washed and dried.

When themes are represented by a collection of appropriate pictures, the vocabulary for these stable, familiar situations can be mounted in thematic displays. Dedicated bathroom, kitchen and fast food restaurant displays can be created for use in those situations. When mounted on walls, on appliances or in racks, these symbols are readily accessible for use by anyone at any time. They can even promote peer interaction!

Even better, the personal picture symbol displays that your partner carries with her at all times remain distinctively hers. She won't have to wade through pictures for "towel", "soap", "bathtub" to get to "movie"!

LET'S REVIEW

Help your partner's augmentative or alternative communication system become her voice.

When your partner is ready for an AAC system the decision to implement this system should be made jointly by your partner and her team.
AAC systems need to be:

Flexible — containing common vocabulary that can be used in any situation

The AAC system should contain vocabulary that enables your partner to participate in a variety of communicative routines such as introducing herself, using greetings and requesting the time. In order to ensure that she has some control in the interaction, it should also contain phrases such as "I'm not done yet" and "Let me do it".

Active — capable of being used purposefully and functionally during interactions

The AAC system is only useful if it is used actively by you, your partner and her friends, peers and family. When it becomes a natural and comfortable part of almost every interaction between your partner and the people with whom she interacts, and when she is using it to speak for herself, you can be sure that it is being used actively.

Individualized — containing vocabulary that serves your partner's unique communicative needs

Vocabulary selection is an ongoing, dynamic process that requires careful observation of your partner's needs and interests before, during and after interactions. Because each partner's needs and interests are unique and ever-changing, vocabulary should be constantly updated and revised.

Respected — viewed and treated as an intrinsic, valuable part of the interaction between your partner and you

The best way to ensure that an AAC system is respected is to give your partner the time she needs to use it successfully, without communicating for her. Keeping the system easily accessible and up to date also demonstrates to your partner that her system is considered important and is respected.

Chapter Seven Create Activities with a Purpose

Until now, you have encouraged your partner to communicate in a natural, incidental way as opportunities arose. You have probably noticed that some situations provide many more opportunities for interaction and sharing of activities than others. In order to provide your partner with as many opportunities as possible to share experiences and to become a participant in the conversations, you will need to create activities with a purpose. Within these activities, you can help him achieve specific communication goals.

Your partner will benefit if you carefully plan how you will use the time you spend together to encourage his communication. First, you have to select some goals — goals that are specific, useful and attainable. Then, your challenge is to create many opportunities throughout the day in which the goal(s) can be modelled for him since he needs frequent exposure to models of the skills he's going to learn before he will try them himself. In addition, he needs to practise using these skills in a variety of situations. Only then can he integrate them into his day-to-day interactions.

In this chapter you will learn to:

- choose appropriate communication goals which are specific, useful and attainable

- involve your partner in activities that will enhance his interaction and learning

- promote communication in a number of environments

- help your partner achieve goals at the next stage of communication

CHOOSE APPROPRIATE COMMUNICATION GOALS

Select communication goals that are:

- specific
- useful
- attainable

Select communication goals that are specific

The more specific you can be in describing your goal, the better are your partner's chances of achieving it. The goal can be a specific sign such as "score", a gesture, such as "cold", an action word such as "hit (the puck)", one more turn in an activity, or learning to communicate for a specific reason (such as asking you to do something for him). The checklists in Chapter 1 and information in this chapter will help you to be specific in your description of goals.

Select communication goals that are useful

A useful goal can be defined as a word, sign, symbol or gestures that would make your partner's efforts to communicate easier, clearer and more informative. The most useful goals are those which your partner wants to say but can't (leaving him and you frustrated) or which would help him participate in activities.

Select communication goals that are attainable

If the goal is appropriate for your partner's level of communication and if it is something he is motivated to learn, then it is attainable.

To individualize communication goals for your partner, ask yourself the following questions:

- Which words, signs or symbols would be most useful and motivating for my partner to learn?
- Which goals involve communication that is a natural part of activities that my partner enjoys?
- For which reasons does my partner not communicate and which of these would enrich his ability to interact with others?
- What has my partner tried to communicate to me that I could not understand, or could only figure out after a period of time?

- What has my partner tried to communicate to me that only one or two other people could understand?
- Which goals best fit my partner's level of communication? What do the checklists in Chapter 1 suggest?
- What do previous speech, language and communication assessments suggest as possible goals?

Examples of individualized and attainable goals are outlined below.

Partners at Level 1

The goal for your partner who responds reflexively, might focus on encouraging him to attend briefly to you or to an interesting object.

Partners at Level 2

At this level, your partner sends messages unintentionally through body language. Thus, the goal here might be focused on creating situations in which he has to approach you or attend to you to get what he wants.

Partners at Level 3

At this level, your partner's communication is intentional. Your goal might be for him to use more conventional behaviours and/or to combine such conventional behaviours. For example, you might encourage your partner to tap you on the arm to get your attention and then reach for something he wants.

Partners at Level 4

At Level 4, your partner can represent ideas and things with individual symbols such as words, pictures or signs. An appropriate goal, therefore, would involve encouraging imitation and then spontaneous use of a new symbol.

Partners at Level 5

At Level 5, your partner is able to combine words into three-word combinations and/or use phrases. Your goals could involve expanding his three-word phrases into four- and five-word phrases and then building phrases into short sentences.

Partners at Level 6

When your partner can speak in sentences, it is helpful for your goals to focus on developing conversational skills so that he learns to use his language appropriately in social situations. Goals could include maintaining the topic, contributing additional information related to the conversation or asking questions. Your partner's speech-language pathologist or other qualified support person is the one who should be able to help you identify and facilitate acquisition of these goals.

REMEMBER . . . When choosing a goal, be realistic. Use the checklists in Chapter 1 together with the information in this chapter to help you. If the goal is too easy or too hard, you'll find out and you can adjust it accordingly.
To facilitate your partner's acquisition of these goals:

- **A**dapt your activities as well as your behaviour; and then
- **A**llow your partner to lead
- **A**dd information that your partner can understand and from which he can learn

Augment your partner's communication, as you learned in Chapter 6, if necessary.

INVOLVE YOUR PARTNER IN ACTIVITIES THAT ENHANCE INTERACTION AND LEARNING

Adapt your activities to accommodate goals for your partner

In Chapters 3 and 4, you learned how to adapt activities as well as your own behaviour to create opportunities for your partner to learn. When planning activities, continue to adapt them so that you:

- make it necessary for your partner to share an item that is part of the activity
- play simple games with your partner that require turn-taking
- respond differently than you normally do in common routines or situations
- respond literally to your partner's communications rather than making assumptions about what he wants
- ask appropriate questions

When such adaptations are implemented throughout the day, you will create many more opportunities to model the communicative goal/s for your partner.

Reduce distractions and engage your partner's attention

To focus your partner's attention, reduce distractions. Gather all necessary materials before starting and put everything else away. Keep the noise level to a minimum. Turn off the TV, radio and dishwasher. If the people nearby aren't otherwise occupied, involve them in what you are doing. **Begin with a favourite activity to attract your partner's attention or to calm him.**

Part of planning any activity involves making sure your partner's attention is engaged. This involves asking yourself the following:

- How can I hook my partner's interest?
- How can I increase my partner's participation and interaction?
- How can I share a focused activity with my partner while allowing him to lead?
- How can I facilitate my partner's communication and language learning within this activity?

Your planned activity will be most productive if both of you are relaxed and ready for it. Don't try to initiate an interaction if your partner is happily absorbed in something else or is upset, distracted or sleepy. And don't start if you are preoccupied with other responsibilities.

A well-chosen activity will usually get and hold your partner's attention, but if he is difficult to engage, try one or a combination of the following suggestions:

- get involved in what he is doing, and gradually redirect him to your planned activity
- invite your partner into the activity
- call his name or say "Look at this"
- show your partner an item involved in the activity
- tempt your partner — get involved in the activity yourself while he is nearby, or invite others into the activity and let your partner see you enjoying yourselves; then wait for him to join you.
- gently turn your partner toward you
- wait for any inattentive or disruptive behaviour to stop
- try again later

Introduce the activity using simple language

When you first introduce the activity, keep your instructions simple. A lot of talking is not necessary. Demonstrating what is involved is often enough to get your partner involved. Once your partner becomes more familiar with the activity, he will be able to concentrate more easily on your language and communication models.

Try something new, but don't abandon the old

If there are activities that you and your partner have never attempted before — like sailing, for instance — try them! Choose a project that seems suited to his general level of development. Who knows? It may be more fun than you think! Sometimes it's a good idea to try something just above your partner's skill level. Without realizing it, you may have underestimated his talents. Of course, if you've overestimated him, you'll soon know!

As your partner progresses to more complicated activities, he won't leave his old skills and interests behind. He will often want to go back to tried-and-true activities. For example, a person who has learned to arrange bouquets of flowers and balloons may still enjoy popping the balloons once in a while. The sense of security your partner gains from something familiar gives him the confidence to try something new.

Respond to your partner's initiations and add information

Try not to become so absorbed with the goal and the activity you've chosen that you don't notice your partner's initiations. If he shows an interest in an equally valid activity or goal, abandon your own agenda and **allow him to lead**. For example, if you are modelling the word "open" and your partner is not interested in imitating the word, you could change the goal to "no" or "don't want." However, if he is distracted by something unproductive, respond to the initiation and then bring him back to the activity you've planned.

When your partner initiates or performs an action within an activity, it may seem that saying "Good work" or "Good, Bob" in response to your partner's efforts is a positive response. However, this kind of response doesn't give him the information he needs and it often ends the conversation. Instead of evaluating him, take advantage of opportunities to make **informative comments** such as "Yes, weeds." "Pull the weeds." "Okay, try again, pull those wwweeds."

Enjoy yourselves!

Choose an activity that you too will enjoy. Your enthusiasm and good humour will rub off on your partner and he will have more fun too. Sometimes it's a good idea to plan ways of involving him in things you enjoy doing. Shopping, building a table, collecting bugs or singing karaoke are rich language-learning experiences!

Your aim is for your partner to enjoy being with you and to have many opportunities to practise his communication. It is important not to push him too hard or to demand too much. Finish the planned activity before your partner tires or loses interest. If necessary, interact for short periods of time, especially at the beginning.

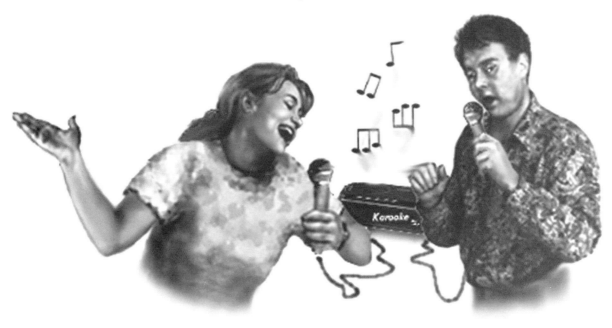

> **REMEMBER . . .** you won't need to plan a new activity every day. People with cognitive delays benefit from lots and lots of repetition, so you will use the same activity many, many times.

PLAN TO PROMOTE COMMUNICATION ACROSS ENVIRONMENTS

Opportunities for communication abound in every aspect of life. Typically, your partner is involved in activities in four broad areas, all of which have the potential for social and functional interaction in varying degrees. Your partner's learning can be greatly enhanced if all of his conversation partners work together on the same goals. This will enable him to transfer his skills to all of the environments in which he spends his time.

• *Home*
Residential settings offer some of the best opportunities for communication because this is usually where your partner feels most comfortable and emotionally available to learn. Many activities take place throughout the day at home. The airwaves are rich with actions, sounds and words which are part of daily routines. Home is where the heart is.

• *Community*
Like any of us, your partner probably spends a lot of time in shopping malls, banks, hospitals, libraries, faith centres, community service groups, at charity

drives, dances, at the movies or in video stores. Depending on where he goes and what he does there, he could have any number of messages to convey to clerks, professionals, customers or any other person he might meet. The community can be a rich source of communication goals.

• Recreation

Most of us spend a lot of time planning activities we enjoy. Recreation implies enjoyment, group socialization and the indulging of personal interests. Interaction is inherent in these recreational activities. Whether you are helping your partner to learn how to play ping-pong or to understand how dating works, goals in the area of recreation lend themselves readily to communication.

• Work

Adult vocational training literally occurs "on the job". Work settings are as varied as the kinds of skills to be learned — from the gift shop to the workshop to the car lot. Learning a trade naturally involves a routine or sequence, a set of new vocabulary and/or a new setting or experience. Verbal and nonverbal communication can enhance your partner's understanding and ability to deal with all of the steps necessary to acquiring these job skills. Work situations can also be a means to furthering his social relationships with his co-workers.

• Educational programs

Many adults with language impairments are involved in literacy or educational programs. In these programs they learn important skills which are needed to function more independently in the community. Opportunities for learning language and communication skills are inherent in many of the activities in this environment.

The formalized planning process involving your partner and his support team is a good place to begin sharing information about communication goals and to co-ordinate your efforts. If it is not possible to get a team together to work on common goals, you can still use these strategies in goal planning. Partners with developmental delays are very good at distinguishing between who is more responsive to them and who is not!

SET GOALS TO HELP YOUR PARTNER MOVE TO THE NEXT STAGE OF COMMUNICATION

On the following pages you will find examples of goals and activities that have arisen in our work in each of these four areas. You, too, can personalize goals in those situations that are unique to you and your partner. If these goals can be encouraged across all settings, you may be surprised at your partner's success!

Encourage non-verbal communication through motor imitation

Activities and interactions can aim at encouraging non-verbal communication at your partner's level. It is easier for fledgling communicators to get their messages across using their body. **Facial expressions and gestures** communicate quite clearly when your partner is very interested in getting that magazine or going for a ride. You might encourage motor imitation of the following actions:

- pointing
- reaching
- tapping
- touching
- looking
- signalling
- gesturing
- pointing + reaching
- eye gaze + vocalization
- pointing + looking
- reaching + gesturing
- touching + signalling
- touching + vocalizing
- showing + reaching
- looking at you then at the desired object

These messages should always be considered in conjunction with the reasons for which your partner communicates (see the checklist "**Why**" your partner communicates on pages 19 and 20). For example, a communication goal might be: "Point to ask for a drink" or "Gesture for help".

Examples of messages your partner at the preverbal stage might want to send using non-verbal means:

Come here	Hello	Want	Don't want	More
Hungry/eat	Cold	Big	Drink	Stop
Phone	Hot	That way	Go out/in	Ride
Visit Mom	Music	Sit with me	Get it	No
Want that one	Up there	Put it in	Put it there	Yes
Sick	Go away	Book/Magazine	Special possessions	

Carolyn enjoys any snack. However, snacks are usually supplied and Carolyn does not need to ask for them. Katie, her facilitator, decided to change this and so she identified reaching in order to request a snack as a goal for Carolyn. The next time they sat down together to share a snack, Katie cut an apple up into several pieces and gave them to Carolyn one piece at a time. After several pieces, Katie waited before giving Carolyn a piece. If, after 15 to 90 seconds Carolyn did not initiate a reach, Katie ate a piece herself. Carolyn caught on and began to initiate reaches — 15 times in 10 minutes!

Margaret is an older woman who does not speak. She has just moved into a group home. Her facilitator, Jan, is involving Margaret in preparing the meal, probably for the first time in Margaret's life! Margaret likes to move things, and Shake'n'Bake™ chicken seemed like the ideal supper choice in which the goal for "shake" could be encouraged. Together Margaret and Jan place prepared chicken pieces into a bag of bread crumbs. Jan instructs Margaret to "Shake, shake, shake!" while modelling a gesture for "shake". Margaret does so easily. This continues as Margaret shakes several pieces of chicken, with Jan modelling the gesture. Then Jan decides to take a turn. While holding the bag, she looks at Margaret and waits, and finally asks, "What should I do?" Margaret shows her what she should do by imitating Jan's shaking gesture!

Encourage the transition from motor to vocal imitation

If your partner doesn't imitate speech sounds, start with non-speech sounds. Encourage your partner to imitate these sounds:

- blowing – such as blowing bubbles, blowing out a candle
- smacking lips – as if enjoying the taste of food
- crying sound
- sneezing or coughing
- animal sounds

Some random sounds, if responded to consistently, can become meaningful in time.

If your partner is beginning to make sounds, you can help him learn to associate a commonly used action with an interesting sound. This will focus his attention on imitating sounds.

Examples of sounds which might be interesting enough for your partner to imitate:

- sound of vacuum cleaner
- "m-m-m" (good), (rub stomach)
- "oops!" (object falling)
- "swish swish" (broom on floor)
- "rat-tat-tat" (typewriter)
- "razzing" sound (tongue vibrating between teeth)
- "bye" and wave
- "bang" (sudden fall)
- "brmm" (car motor sound)

Christine communicates at Level 2. She is always vocalizing, whether sitting alone or in a group. No one responds to the sounds she makes since the sounds don't seem to be directed at anyone in particular. Her facilitator, Jane, decided to work on making Christine's vocalizations more purposeful.

Jane knows that Christine enjoys one-to-one attention, drinks and walks outside. She decides to ask the question, "Do you want to go outside?" before opening the door for Christine and to wait for Christine to respond by making a sound.

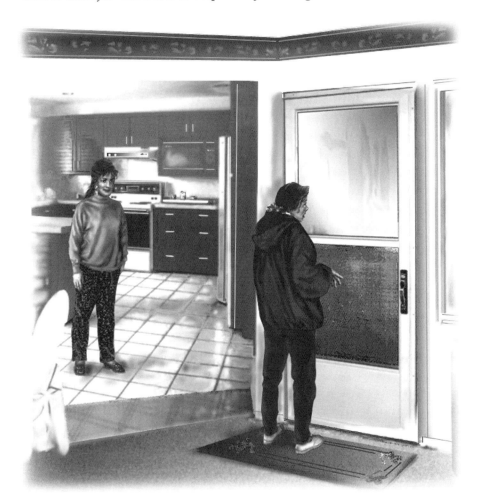

Christine wants to go outside, but before Jane opens the door for her, she will help her learn to use sounds to send a clear message.

When Christine approaches the door, Jane walks over to her, puts her hand on the door handle and asks, "Do you want to go outside?" As soon as Christine vocalizes, Jane says, "Yes, outside", nods and pushes the door open. This simple plan enables Christine to grasp the connection between her vocalizations and the door opening. 🌿

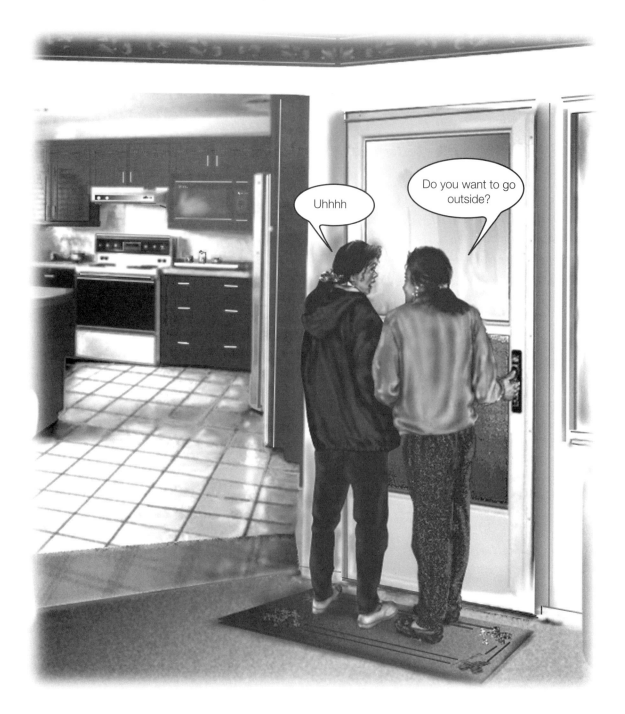

Jane opens the door only after Christine responds to her question by making a sound. This way, Christine learns that her sounds are the key to getting Jane to open the door.

Encourage single-word vocabulary in everyday activities

If your partner is beginning to use part-words, words, pictures or signs, there are many ways to expand his vocabulary during everyday activities.

The following lists are provided as examples of vocabulary goals that can be encouraged at home, during academic and recreational activities or during work in the community. The sections of the chapter contain stories which describe activities in which goals are modelled, and which demonstrate their eventual use by the partner. Here you can apply all of your skills in waiting, using signals and appropriate questions. You will know if your partner is ready and willing to use the selected goal when he begins to use it himself. Keep the questions at the beginning of this chapter in front of you. *Be open and sensitive to your partner.* Who knows, he may develop an acceptable goal that is different from yours!

Promote vocabulary during personal care activities

Nouns			*Action Words*			
sock	comb	lipstick	brush	comb	wash	give
pyjamas	shirt	pants	pull	wet	squeeze	shake
shampoo	soap	dress	blow	stop	rinse	feel
nylons	shoes	eye shadow	help	reach	hear	pick up
mascara	cologne	shaver	pour	wipe	cut	shave
dryer	braid	deodorant	hit	rub	stop	buy
head	hand	legs	run	walk	sleep	go
eyes	hair	nose	push	throw	roll	sit
pony tail	coat	toothbrush	tie	drink	see	open
toothpaste	cup	water	fall	stand	shower	close
cupboard	bandage	scissors	put	gimme	fold	break
bubbles	tangles	haircut	pull	carry	hurt	find
purse	scarf	sweater	dress	choose	take	wear
nail polish	bath	cream	streak	dye	braid	tease

REMEMBER . . . When choosing vocabulary, remind yourself of the difference between expressive and receptive language. Typically, most people **understand more than they express**. You can use a wider range of vocabulary when facilitating your partner's understanding of words than when you are trying to expand his expressive vocabulary.

*B*ill *is involved in a janitorial crew. His facilitators and job support worker feel it is important for him to learn the word "wash". Several activities throughout the day are adapted so Bill and his facilitators spend time doing them together. These include washing dishes, clothes, windows, floors, the dog, Bill's hair and so on. Facilitators describe and explain what is happening throughout the activity, with special emphasis and repetition on the word, "wash".*

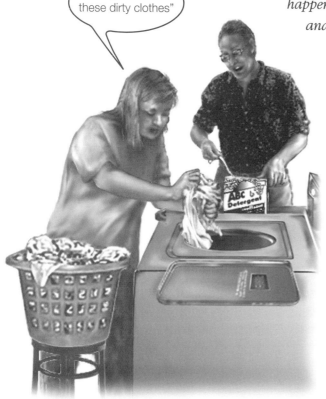

"Okay, let's **wash** these dirty clothes"

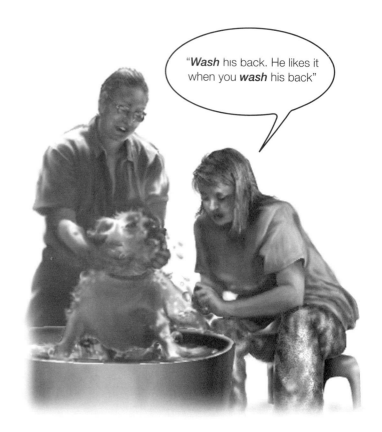

"**Wash** his back. He likes it when you **wash** his back"

Bill is learning the word "wash" from hearing his facilitator model it in many different situations.

One day Jim, one of Bill's facilitators, is washing the dishes while Bill is drying them. Jim picks up a dish, holds it just above the water and looks at Bill expectantly, waiting. At first, Jim has to model the word, "Wash", and when Bill catches on, he uses the word for every dirty dish!

Promote vocabulary around the kitchen

Nouns			*Action Words*			
dish	spoon	fork	wash	cook	cut	knead
knife	spatula	bowl	mix	grind	whip	squeeze
pot	pan	griddle	fry	boil	bake	turn on
fryer	crockpot	plate	warm	heat	put	open
cup	glass	tea	pour	close	blend	peel
coffee	favourite foods		throw	toss	grate	crush
refrigerator	stove	milk	zap	nuke	wash	sort
microwave	oven	kettle	shop	buy	drink	eat
blender	table	shake	invite	perk	clean	mop
dishwasher	soap	cleanser	wipe	rub	fall	more
garbage	apron	placemat	wear	set	want	
dessert	supper	breakfast				

*T*im has cerebral palsy and cannot speak. He is very friendly and initiates frequently using gestures. A picture symbol system has been developed for him and although he is able to use the system, he does not use it. His facilitator, Mark, takes a closer look at the vocabulary included in Tim's system and observes that much of it is not functional. When Mark spends time with Tim making a cup of tea, he adds more useful vocabulary, such as "water", "cup" and "milk". After a few models of these words, Tim begins using them as requests himself!

Promote vocabulary while doing housework

Nouns			*Action Words*			
vacuum	duster	mop	dust	mop	clean	wipe
bed	carpet	floor	make	fold	rub	scrub
wall	lamp	table	spray	wash	dry	shine
cleanser	bucket	sponge	wax	polish	pull	open
box	cupboard	shelf	reach	close	need	more
paper towel	laundry	softener	gone	shake	brush	vacuum
broom	dustpan	sink	feel	buy	push	carry
			come	put	see	give
			hang	tear	sweep	

*V*ince lives in a group home and shares responsibility with his mates for keeping the house clean. His facilitator, Todd, wants to boost Vince's gestural repertoire of action words, and in this instance he is concentrating on the concept "tear".

Vince and Todd are going around the house cleaning all the glass and polished surfaces. While Vince sprays the surface with glass cleaner, Todd dispenses the paper towels so Vince can clean the glass. Every time Vince needs a sheet, Todd models the gesture for "tear".

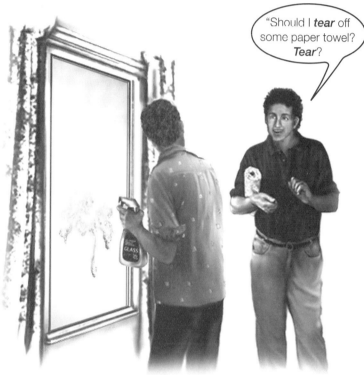

"Should I *tear* off some paper towel? *Tear*?"

By pairing the word and the gesture "tear" many, many times…

After several models of the word and gesture for "tear" over a couple of sessions, Todd begins to wait expectantly for Vince to initiate the request. Sure, enough, Vince uses the gesture for "tear" that he has seen modelled so many times!

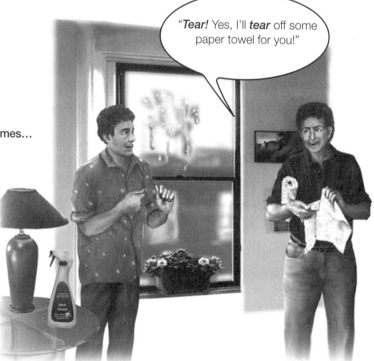

"*Tear!* Yes, I'll *tear* off some paper towel for you!"

… Todd helps Vince learn to use the gesture himself.

Another action word that Todd focuses on is the gesture for "spray". Todd and Vince switch roles with Todd cleaning the surfaces and Vince dispensing the paper towels. Prior to squirting glass cleaner on the surface, Todd makes sure that Vince is paying attention and he then models the gesture for "spray". He does this each time he cleans a surface. After several models, Todd begins to wait expectantly. Well, you get the picture. Todd has to signal first, by placing his fingers in the beginning position of the gesture. After several turns at this, Vince begins to gesture by lifting his index finger! Todd accepts this as an acceptable attempt at communication, and continues to model the more correct form throughout subsequent activities in the hope that Vince's gesture will become more accurate. ❧

Promote vocabulary while working in the yard

Nouns			*Action Words*			
plants	flower	grass	plant	cut	mow	weed
mud/soil	mower	hoe	rake	trim	water	turn
rake	can	seed	grow	sweep	throw	
composter	tree	bush	decorate			

Gilles *is part of a maintenance crew. His facilitators are working on increasing his single-word vocabulary, especially job-related words. One of the words which his facilitator Vern has targeted is "seed", and he plans to help Gilles learn this word when they plant flowers and a vegetable garden in the spring. During the planting activity, Vern hands Gilles the seeds one by one, modelling the word "seed" while Gilles plants each one. After five to 10 models, Vern holds back the seed, and waits expectantly for Gilles to attempt the word. To his surprise, Gilles begins to use the word "seed" consistently to request each one.*

*Gilles' facilitators continue to be interested in increasing his opportunities to initiate, communicate and develop vocabulary. They select another goal — the word "in". They decide to help Gilles learn this word during everyday chores as well as during seasonal ones. One activity in which they model this word repetitively is raking leaves in the fall. When the leaves have been gathered, Gilles holds open a large bag so Vern can drop them in. Every time Vern drops some leaves in the bag, he uses the word "**in**" in various ways. He says, "**In** the bag.", "Should I put them **in**?", "There they are — **in** the bag. **In**."*

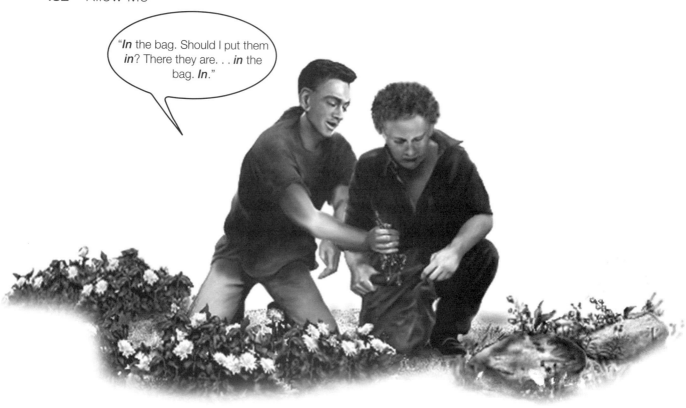

"*In* the bag. Should I put them *in*? There they are. . . *in* the bag. *In*."

Vern uses the word "in" four times as he puts the leaves in the bag, making it much easier for Gilles to learn the word.

When Vern and Gilles arrive at the composter, they do not simply dump all the leaves inside. Instead, during this teaching period, Vern takes some leaves out of the bag and places them in the composter, once again modelling the word "in" each time he drops some leaves into the composter. When he begins to wait expectantly, holding the leaves above the composter but not dropping them in, Gilles surprises Vern by saying, "in".

Promote vocabulary in the community

Nouns			*Action Words*			
bank	store	bus	buy	ride	take	swim
gym	money	taxi	order	phone	pull	push
cart	house	lights	stop	go	open	close
door	car	cab	park	pray	serve	tell
church/synagogue/mosque		stand	sit	read	borrow	float
library	museum	ticket	camp	build	make	walk
boat	camp	park	put	drive	run	fly
shops	tree	street	drive	paint	turn	wait
airplane	restaurant					

*R*obert is very vocal but non-verbal. He uses gestures and sounds to get his messages across but he is extremely difficult to understand. He can use picture symbols to communicate but he rarely does so. Robert is aware of money and what it is used for, so his facilitator, Emily, decides to focus on teaching him how to use the picture symbol for "money". The picture symbol for money is posted in various places where Robert might need to dispense money: the kitchen, the office and his bedroom. Whenever Robert needs more cash, Emily dispenses it one bill or coin at a time, pointing to the picture each time she says the word. Then one day, Robert takes Emily to the picture and points to it himself, quite spontaneously!

This time Emily is working with Robert to encourage him to learn how to use the symbol for "open". Several activities lend themselves well to modelling the word, particularly cooking. While Robert pours and stirs, Emily models use of the picture and the word "open." She says, "**Open** the can.", "The bag is **open**.", "Let's **open** the box." Then it is Robert's turn to open containers, and some are very difficult to open. He doesn't know how to use a can opener and he can't open some of the bags, which are sealed very tightly. Emily has to interpret his intent, "Open?" while pointing to the picture. Once again, Robert catches on. With Emily's help, Robert continues to learn how to use this word in many different contexts, like opening doors, presents and drink boxes. 🌸

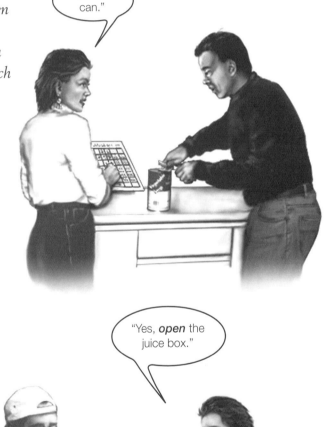

"**Open** the can."

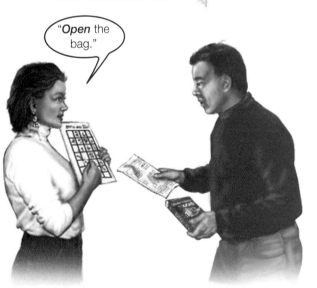

"**Open** the bag."

. . Robert is learning how many things can be opened . . .

"Yes, **open** the juice box."

Promote vocabulary during recreational activities

Nouns			*Action Words*			
game	camp	fire	paint	play	dance	walk
blanket	sweater	scarf	crochet	knit	sew	glue
scissors	craft	tape	tape	cut	colour	staple
pen	pencil	markers	write	make	build	mold
wool	pattern	music	sing	camp	sit	carve
paintbrush	carve	wood	watch	run	swing	hit
baseball	bat	ball	throw	catch	jump	roll
golf	pool	water	swim	stroke	pitch	dive
tape recorder	radio	listen	read	fall	want	fish
tent	trip	holiday	fly	put	row	hook
fishing pole	boat	racket	float	sail	blow	reach
worm	fish	saw	hammer	march	sweep	clean
sports of any type		TV	pass	skate	wrestle	tickle
balloon	Bingo	hockey	match	shoot	hug	
camera	picture	collection				

Promote vocabulary on the job

It may be harder to share activities with your partner in this setting, since you may work with several other partners. However, if your language is geared to his level and focus of interest and activity, your language models will be useful to him. Just remember to keep your goals **specific, useful and attainable.**

Nouns			*Action Words*			
hammer	nail	screw	saw	hit	sand	package
bag	jig	box	put	bag	stack	assemble
machine	button	line	press	tie	seal	tear
pottery	tool	paint	paint	fold	count	carry
table	workshop	job	fall	break	wash	stock
tip	glasses	clean	dust	sweep	take	serve
shovel	wood	hedge	trim	cut	mow	plant
garden	clay	oven	bake	weed	water	cook
mud/soil	bucket	brush	scrub	spray	wipe	clear
paper	folder	plastic	wrap	stuff	staple	open
newspaper	flyer	cart	deliver	sell	pull	throw
garbage	garage	meals	squeeze	twist	stamp	price
photocopy	office	mail	stretch	copy	bring	drink
coffee	break time	apron	split	shovel	rake	
leaves	grass	mower				
store	counter	clerk				

*H*elen is working at a local convenience store. She knows what she wants to say, and is able to use signs and gestures at a one- to two-word level. She has a picture symbol system as a back-up device for those who cannot understand her. Helen has the potential to expand her vocabulary. One of her tasks is to price products using a price tag dispenser. One of the obvious signs she can learn to use is the sign for "price". This task provides Melanie, her job support worker, with hundreds of opportunities to model and encourage the use of this sign. In this task, roles can be easily switched so Melanie is able to model the sign between 10 and 100 times while Helen prices products. When they switch roles, Melanie waits expectantly for Helen to instruct her to put on the price tag before she will price each product. At first, Helen urges her on with a gesture. But Melanie begins to expect more from Helen and, after a few more models, Helen begins to use the sign. It's not perfect, but it's clear enough!

*C*arol is beginning work in an office where she does a lot of stapling. She is an early Level 3 communicator, but her motivation to communicate is relatively low. Her job coach, Ted, wants to encourage her to initiate using a gesture. One of the activities Ted has adapted is a collating task, which involves several copies of a booklet being stapled. Ted and Carol share the stapler, with Ted passing the stapler back and forth between them while making comments such as "I want the **stapler**.", "It's your turn to have the **stapler**.", "Do you want the **stapler**?", "Look, my book is **stapled**." Once Carol becomes accustomed to this routine, Ted begins to hold onto the stapler very briefly as Carol reaches for it. At first, this discourages Carol from taking the stapler. However, when Ted reassures her, Carol takes it from him very, very slowly. Ted increases his expectation that Carol do a little bit more to get the stapler from him. He pulls back just a little bit more, making her reach for it and look at him when he doesn't give it to her immediately. Ted responds to every subtle attempt from Carol to get the stapler. Over time, Carol reaches for the stapler and looks at Ted without hesitation, proving that patience is often the key ingredient to encouraging successful communication.

Promote vocabulary in an educational environment

Nouns			*Action Words*			
pen	pencil	paper	write	draw	push	pull
computer	letter	cheque	ride	clean	shake	cut
button	key	story	fall	count	dial	measure
telephone	brochure	book	work	read	ride	sign
classroom	name	teacher	tell	use	plan	see
time	bus	lunch	eat	dress	get	change
bank	school	math	stop	go	start	walk
trip	friend	seat	climb	sit	stand	wipe
board	chalk	eraser	guess	weigh	pour	mix
glue	wood	paint	paint	glue	stick	sort
pictures	game	box	match	open	close	shoot
desk	floor	stairs	blow	copy	trace	more
paper clip	stapler	test	staple	clip	stuff	fold
binder	folder	numbers	turn	twist	bend	hang

Riva is John's teacher. They are working on matching skills, and John's task is to cut out matching pictures and mount them. Riva is working on two specific goals: comprehension of the concept "match", and expressive use of the sign for "cut". She uses the word "match" in a variety of ways: "Yes, these cups **match** — they look the same.", "Do the animals **match**?", "This one has long ears and this one doesn't — no, they do not **match**." Riva and John share responsibility for cutting out pictures that match, and the scissors are passed between them. Riva models the sign for "cut" every time she wants to use the scissors, and every time John needs to use the scissors. She also describes what they are doing, and asks John to think beyond the here and now by asking, "What else do we **cut**? We **cut** hair. We can **cut** sandwiches. Did you **cut** your finger?"

After a few sessions and several models Riva signals to encourage John to use the sign himself. However, John is not yet ready, so Riva goes back to modelling the sign, labelling and describing. She knows that John is slower at learning. She is patient, persistent and creative at using the sign at every opportunity. She knows that eventually it will pay off! ✿

Include other word types in your goals

Adjectives		*Social Words*		*Location*		*Emotion-related*
hot	all gone	oh-oh	no	here	out	sad
more	dirty	hi/hello	enough	down	there	loving
my/mine	clean	bye	yes	in	up	happy
big	broken	this/that	okay	on	under	darn/shoot
wet	nice	hey	fine	below	on top	mad
cold	on/off	sorry		between		
soft	sharp	sticky				

Encourage your partner to use two-word phrases

Once your partner has learned, and begins to use the names of objects, actions, people and locations, he is ready to begin stringing words and ideas together.

Here are some examples of common combinations you can begin to model and teach:

Phrases using common verbs

				Location phrases	
Want juice	Want home	Want coffee	Sit down	On table	Fall down
Gimme ball	Gimme pop	Gimme book	Jump up	Walk here	Book there
Wash hands	Wash hair	Wash Spot	In cupboard	Go out	On floor
Go home	Go out	Go away	Slide down	Come here	In bed

Action plus object phrases

			Descriptive phrases	
Throw ball	Eat apple	Brush teeth	Big ball	Cowboy hat
Push door	Wipe table	Kiss baby	More drink	Light on
Wash hands	Shake hand	Paint pictures	Wet soap	TV on
Blow bubble	Button coat	Peel potatoes	No bed	My car/my dog
Open door	Tie shoes	Pour milk	Hot light	Hot stove
Read book	Clap hands	Squirt water	All gone soup	Dirty face
Drink juice	Help me	Ride car	Box empty	
Go toilet				

Noun/pronoun plus action phrases

Car go	You stand	We walk	You paint
Knife cuts	I write	Sally dance	Horse ride
Computer prints	Door open/close	Cars crash	Plant fall
Music plays			

Encourage your partner to use three-word phrases

Once your partner is using two-word phrases consistently, he can begin learning three-word phrases and sentences.

Noun-verb-object phrases

I want coffee	I see them	I like hugs
I want books	I see rain	I like music
I want more	I see Cindy	I like painting
I throw ball	Mark hit me	Man ride bike
Dad push saw	Boy watch TV	You hide shoe
You pour juice	I cut paper	I find shoe
I eat cereal	Karen paint picture	You hug me

Phrases with location added

Dish on table	Plant fall down	I go toilet	Toss bag here
Talk on phone	Put spoon there	Knock on door	We go home
Put shirt on	Take shoes off	Pull pants up	You go to bed
Hide bag under chair	Put soap in water		

Phrases using descriptive words

Comb your hair	Want a red ball	Turn on the music
Want orange juice	Want more juice	Look, a big truck
Boat goes fast	See glasses	My foot hurts
Buy new shoes	Wash my hands	Ice is cold!
Your dress is pretty	Comb my hair	Eat two cookies

Introduce game vocabulary

If your partner can learn how to take part in games, whether cards or spectator sports, it may be helpful to teach him how he can take part. Below is a list of suggestions for game talk.

I won	Roll the dice	Pass	Your deal
My/your turn	What a hand	You go first	You're cheating
Shuffle the cards	Deal me in	I'm out	Check him
That's my man	I need it	Pick one up	Put one down
We're losing	Do you have...?	Game's over	Throw away
Go this way	Pick a card	Nice shot	I'll knock you off
Hit that ball!	He struck out	Way to go!	Let's play again

USE THE 4 "I"S TO PLAN, IMPLEMENT AND EVALUATE YOUR GOALS IN SHARED ACTIVITIES

Once you have identified the opportunities in your partner's life for communication and you have selected goals that arise from these opportunities, consider how you will implement an action plan to encourage your partner to learn these goals. The 4 "I" Action Plan (see pages 140 and 141) will help you to plan activities that:

- are **Interesting**
- require your partner to **Initiate**
- are **Interactive**
- provide **Informatiom** at his level

When planning how to help your partner achieve a goal, you deliberately create and foster an enriched learning environment that will offer frequent opportunities for him to communicate. Earlier in the chapter, you read how you can engage your partner's attention, the importance of making sure that activities are interactive and informative as well as how to plan for success. If your models are appropriate to your partner's communication level, over time he will begin to use them (however imperfectly) and you can begin to expect more advanced kinds of messages from him.

If you feel that your partner is making little or no progress, ask yourself these questions:

- Is the language goal too difficult? (If so, can you find a slightly easier step for him to learn first or should you spend more time on preliminary skills such as turn-taking?)
- Is the activity set up in such a way that your partner can initiate?
- Are you responding to your partner's efforts to communicate?
- Can you plan your interaction for a different time or a different place? (Is he hungry or tired? Would he work better in a different room or table?)
- Does your partner really understand what you want him to do? (If not, how can you better get his attention? How can you simplify your language and add gestures?)
- Is the language goal you have chosen too easy? (If so, what goal might be more appropriate?)
- Is the activity you've planned interesting, geared to your partner's skills and language level, and is it enjoyable?

Help Your Partner Achieve
,oals

Name: _____

_____

_____

.vity: _____

.1e activity should be **INTERESTING.**

Plan an activity that is interesting and relevant from your partner's perspective, and that is based on something he can relate to.

_____

_____

Post-activity Evaluation:

What worked or did not work to attract and hold his attention?

_____

_____

2. The activity should allow your partner to **INITIATE.**

How will you allow him to initiate and take an active role in directing the activity?

_____

_____

How will you encourage him to be aware of others in the environment?

_____

_____

Post-activity Evaluation:

How active was your partner in the activity? Is there anything you can try next time to encourage him to take the lead and initiate more often?

_____

_____

3. The activity should be **INTERACTIVE.**

How can you adapt the activity to ensure that there is ongoing interaction between the two of you?

_____

_____

How can you adapt the activity so your partner can clearly send his message to you, even if he doesn't do this intentionally?

_____

_____

How can you adapt the activity so your partner can participate to the best of his ability?

_____

_____

Post-activity Evaluation:

What worked to maintain your partner's participation in the activity and in communicating with you? What didn't work?

_____

_____

4. The activity should allow you to provide **INFORMATION.**

   How can you add information to your partner's messages? How will you respond to his messages in ways that help him learn better ways of communicating?

   _____

   _____   _____

   Post-activity Evaluation:

   List some of your partner's messages and how you responded to them.

   _____

   _____

   Do you need to adjust your responses in any way to make them easier to understand or to keep your partner engaged?

   _____

   _____

   Do you need to adjust your vocabulary goals?

   _____

   _____

   ## General Evaluation of Goals

   At the end of the week, look over your records and make a summary using the following guidelines.

   Have there been any changes in what your partner and you say or do? Specify. _____

   _____

   _____

   What is working well in the activity/ies?

   _____

   _____

   Is there something you would like to change?

   _____

   _____

.MBER . . . Helping people develop communication skills isn't as ...ghtforward as baking a cake or building a bookshelf. There isn't just a ...gle method.

...he necessary ingredients and cooking time vary for each person. What we offer are basic guidelines and, with practice, you will find the recipe that works best for an individual partner. You'll discover what he responds to and what he turns away from, what helps him learn and what doesn't.

Trust your own instincts.

Detailed Table of Contents